Child health maintenance

A GUIDE TO CLINICAL ASSESSMENT

Child health maintenance

A GUIDE TO CLINICAL ASSESSMENT

PEGGY L. CHINN, R.N., Ph.D.

Professor of Nursing,
School of Nursing, Wright State University,
Dayton, Ohio

CYNTHIA J. LEITCH, R.N., Ph.D.

Assistant Professor, School of Nursing,
Community Health Care Systems, University of Washington,
Seattle, Washington

SECOND EDITION

The C. V. Mosby Company

ST. LOUIS • TORONTO • LONDON   1979

SECOND EDITION

Printed in the United States of America

The C. V. Mosby Company
11830 Westline Industrial Drive, St. Louis, Missouri 63141

Library of Congress Cataloging in Publication Data

Chinn, Peggy L   1941-
    Child health maintenance.

    Bibliography: p.
    1.   Pediatric nursing.   2.   Child development—
Testing.   3.   Children—Care and hygiene.
I.   Leitch, Cynthia J., 1933-   joint author.
II.   Title.   [DNLM: 1.   Child care.   2.   Child
development.   3.   Child health services.
4.   Growth—In adolescence.   5.   Pediatric nursing.
WY159 C5395c]
RJ245.C48   1979   610.73′62   78-11964
ISBN 0-8016-0949-6

GW/CB/CB   9   8   7   6   5   4   3   2   1   03/D/340

Preface

This clinical guide is intended to fulfill two basic purposes. First, it provides a learning guide for students who are acquiring the ability to perform a comprehensive health assessment; second, it provides a resource of information and materials that are frequently needed in the actual provision of health care to children. This guide is not intended as a comprehensive text, nor is it the purpose of the book to present the background knowledge that is needed to conduct the assessment outlined here. The scope and depth of assessment presented may well extend beyond the skill and ability of the student or the practicing nurse. The guide is intended to stimulate further learning and experience in those areas of assessment where knowledge or skill is lacking. Users may modify the suggestions included according to the situation and their present stage of ability.

Provided herein is basic information regarding developmental differences that are observed throughout childhood from birth through adolescence, along with an indication of deviations that may occur and implications for health care. Furthermore, information that is commonly needed to implement a plan of care is included in accessible cross-reference form. It is anticipated that through the practice of assessment with a wide range of children, the student will develop knowledge and sensitivity that surpass the scope of this reference. Although this tool is not intended to become a "crutch," it is anticipated that it will remain a valuable reference for some of the details of growth and development that are not practically committed to memory. In addition, such material as the list of community resources, normative growth data, laboratory values, nutrition information, and conversion tables for weights and measures will continue to be useful for clinicians. The user is urged to make personally meaningful notes to expand the use of the guide for the individual situation.

It will be noted that emphasis is consistently placed on the maintenance of health and identification of the health needs of children. Although one purpose of health assessment is to find conditions that require medical attention, the emphasis here is placed on the purpose of identifying the health needs of children. Where specialist referral or consultation is indicated, the specific medical, dental, educational, social, or counseling problems are referred to appropriate care workers. The primary health care worker continues to serve the child and his or her family according to the identified primary health needs and the ability of the individual clinician.

Detailed discussion of each area of assessment outlined in this guide is presented in the text, *Child Health Maintenance: Concepts in Family-Centered Care*. The user is referred

v

to this text, other textbooks, and current journals for expansion of the knowledge, skill, and theory that are needed to provide comprehensive health care for children and families.

Appreciation is expressed to each of those who used the first edition of this guide and who offered valuable suggestions for revision. Particular appreciation is extended to Cheryl Hundley, R.N., B.S., who designed the infant, child, and play assessment tools included in the guide, and to Patsy Kaiser, R.N., M.S., and Donna Kem, R.N., C.N.M., M.S., for granting permission to adapt their family assessment tool for use in this guide.

Peggy L. Chinn

Contents

1 Introduction, 1

2 Assessment of physical competency, 10

3 Assessment of learning and thought, social, and inner competencies, 38

4 Norms and standards for nursing assessment and intervention, 51

5 Criteria for hospitalization and home care, 86

6 Management of common illness in childhood, 91

7 Sexual function and family planning, 103

8 Guidelines to nutritional assessment, 108

9 Community and national resources, 121

10 Assessment tools and case audit guide, 128

Appendix: Conversion tables and equivalents, 152

References and additional resources, 157

CHAPTER 1

Introduction

COMMUNICATION WITH FAMILIES AND CHILDREN

Perhaps the most important skill involved in health care of children and families is the skill of communication. The tasks performed and the information gathered in rendering health care become meaningful and relevant by the process that occurs between the health care worker, the child, and the family. These processes are depicted in Fig. 1-1. In this diagram the child and the significant adult are represented as overlapping, separate units, because each shares overlapping concerns, and communication from each significant person involved in a particular child health problem is essential in formulating reliable and relevant judgments. The nurse and the child/adult units are seen as separate human entities within an encompassing sensory encounter transaction circle. Each sends the other some kind of communicative message through action, verbal message, or inquiry. This is represented as a solid arrow in the direction of the message sent. The person receiving the message then gives some form of feedback, or validation, indicating receipt of the message. This is represented as a broken arrow in the direction of the feedback sent, signifying the fact that this message may not always be sent or perceived in a totally accurate manner. Sometimes the communication sent is inadequate; at other times there is an inadequacy in the perception of the message by the receiver or in the perception of the feedback.

When the health care worker uses this process skillfully, a valuable transaction process of validation, reevaluation, and reciprocal relationship is formulated, enabling the nurse and the child/adult to each continually participate in the formulation of goals to be achieved. Within the framework of sensory encounter and transaction, the health care worker, specifically, is executing the acts of skilled judgment based on assessment, intervention, and management. The child and the adult remain an integral part of the process through the transaction and communication processes that are ongoing and continuous.

The interview

The child/adult interview presents a special challenge, because information must be obtained from both the child and significant adults who provide nurturance and care. Subjective information from either the child or the adult may contain consistencies or inconsistencies and may or may not be corroborated by observation of actual behavior. Where conflicting information emerges, value should be placed equally on each source of information, and the underlying source of the conflict becomes the focus of the health care worker.

Developing skill in interviewing parents and

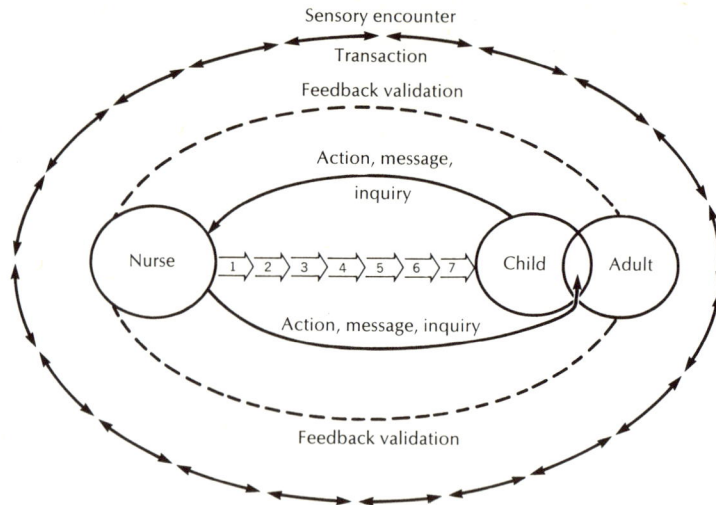

Fig. 1-1. Process of child nursing care. The seven components of nursing action are (1) identify values and goals to be attained, (2) identify structure, process, and outcome standards and criteria for goal attainment, (3) measure degree of attainment of selected standards and criteria, (4) interpret available data, (5) identify alternative nursing actions, (6) select the course of action, and (7) implement the course of action. Evaluation of the nursing process is accomplished by review and audit of each component in comparison with professional standards of practice.

children requires a great deal of practice and patience. The approach used in any given situation depends on the developmental level of the child and the adult. An encounter with a health care worker often arouses emotional undertones, because a child who is not totally healthy is considered as evidence, in most societies, of poor performance on the part of the caretaker. In reality this may not be the case, but our traditional approaches and health care system reinforce this societal assumption. Defensiveness, fear, and uncertainty can be hidden but are real barriers to receiving reliable and valuable information, even if the child is essentially well.

Thus the important factor in interviewing becomes the process and not the exact content. Certain areas of content, such as features of pregnancy, delivery, developmental milestones, and signs of any present problems or health needs, should be included. The health care worker is interested in eliciting content that adds meaningfully to the process of identifying needs for the maintenance and promotion of health for this specific child.

The health care worker is an advocate for the child. The interview should be employed as an important screening device for problems of physical and emotional health. Questions that are directed toward uncovering adequacies and inadequacies in the family-child relationships are particularly important for the child's protection and benefit. The following summary of "do's and don'ts" is designed to help in developing an effective and nonthreatening approach to exploring the child's world:

Do ask	Don't ask
How do you manage?	What do you do with Johnny while you work?
Tell me about your childhood.	Did your parents beat you?
Where did you grow up?	Were they mean to you?
What was it like?	
Tell me about Johnny when he was a baby.	Did you have problems with Johnny when he was a baby?
Tell me about Johnny when he first walked (talked, went to preschool, and so on).	At what age did Johnny walk?
What was it like for the two of you?	

Most adults do not remember specific dates or cannot recite the exact nature of the problems a child may have. It is important to ask general, nondirective questions first, picking up as many clues as possible; then ask for specific information after an atmosphere of acceptance has been demonstrated.

Active listening

Active listening is a counseling technique that may be used in regard to several problems identified in the assessment. This technique involves listening to the report of the parent or child, then reflecting back on your own perception of what has been said or implied, always responding to the effect messages as well as the content. For example:

MOTHER (in a distressed tone of voice): I honestly don't know what to do about these temper tantrums. I think I get it figured out, then he has a tantrum and all my plans go to pot. I end up screaming and spanking him. My husband is even worse.

NURSE: I know this is terribly frustrating. You seem to be thinking and planning what you are going to do about the next tantrum, and then you find it doesn't work (mother nods). Apparently this is just as frustrating for your husband.

MOTHER: Yes, only he gets even more upset and blames me for not being able to handle the child.

NURSE: The two of you have a difference of opinion over how to manage?

MOTHER (calmer now): Oh no, not really. We have really tried to plan what we're going to do together. But I'm with Billy all day, and my husband can't understand why our plans fall apart.

NURSE: Being with a child all day is hard, and I can tell that you resent being blamed for the problem continuing (mother nods). Tell me about your plans that haven't seemed to work.

Here the nurse is eliciting real information. The mother has an opportunity to clear up a misunderstanding the nurse seems to have about husband-wife conflict. Her anxiety and distress are acknowledged and begin to dissipate. Arbitrary advice-giving is avoided by the nurse. Once the mother's approaches are understood, the two can work together toward a meaningful, helpful resolution.

The child

Giving periodic attention to the child, either through play or by eliciting active involvement in the interview, creates a relaxed, nonstructured, accepting atmosphere. In communication with children of all ages, the following general principles lead to development of rapport and meaningful responses.

Use a quiet, confident tone of voice when you speak to children. If you speak softly to children they will pay more attention to you than if you raise your voice.

Give your directions in as few words as possible, and make them specific, not general. Children who are just learning to go to the toilet regularly will understand if you say to them, "Toilet time now," and hold out your hand for them to come. They are more likely to say "no" if you say, "Well, you have played a long time, you should go to the toilet. Come, we'd better hurry." They are confused by too many words.

Give children plenty of time. Children often resist if they feel that you are hurrying them. Perhaps they have not had time to park a truck where they wanted to leave it. We can respect their purposes without encouraging them to "stall." If they think of one thing after another to delay coming into the examining room, the nurse can explain: "It's time to come to the other room now. As soon as you finish that puzzle you need to come." Then when the child finishes, gently and quietly take his or her hand and begin to talk about a game you will be playing in the other room.

Make your suggestions positive ones. Tell children what you want them to do rather than what you don't want them to do. The easiest way to do this is to avoid the use of the word "don't." You will have better results if you say, "You need to sit on the chair," instead of, "Don't stand on the chair."

Interest children in positive behavior. Help children by making desirable behavior seem interesting and fun. "Can you pretend you are the tallest person in the world? Show me how big that is!" You may help children by giving them something to look forward to if they do their part by saying, "As soon as you have washed your hands, you may listen through my stethoscope."

Encourage children to be independent in taking care of themselves and in their play. Give them enough time to get into their own clothes. Give them only as much help as they really seem to need. Address the major portion of your conversation and interview to school-age children, not their parents. Encourage their own expression of their needs, feelings, and memory of past health and health care practices.

Children should be warned just in advance as to what is going to happen next. "When you finish getting dressed, I will test your eyes." Once you have given warning that a thing is to happen, follow through with it. Fearful procedures should be approached with confidence and executed quickly but with a brief warning. "It is time for your shot now. It will hurt a minute and then be over." Give the shot quickly; then without delay comfort the child with physical contact, encouraging the parent to do the same. Notice the brief, honest recognition of the fact of pain. The child will be hurt and angry but learns to trust honest predictions.

Enlist children in problem-solving situations. Your success will increase if children, regardless of age, understand their part in solving a problem. If, for instance, the child has pinworms, approach him by saying, "John, we are giving you some medicine to get rid of the bugs that have made your bottom itchy. These bugs sometimes come from chewing things that aren't for eating. Can you think of some things that you like to chew that aren't for eating?" Continue the dialogue in such a manner that the child "discovers" the problem and is able to identify a part of the solution. Or, if a child is older, he or she might also be asked to provide a definition of the problem. The overweight 9-year-old might be asked, "Tell me what you think about the problem."

Use knowledge of children's developmental stages in making the initial approach. Infants who have not yet experienced a separation anxiety respond positively to physical handling. Loud noises and sudden movement are frightening, but infants respond to physical cuddling and close social contact.

During early childhood, play is of utmost importance. After separation anxiety has occurred, an indirect approach using play will often entice young children to make their own approach to strange adults. For example, the adult is stacking blocks or moving a truck around the table with no direct attention to the child.

The young child will watch cautiously for a few minutes and then gradually begin to join the game. Direct interaction can then be comfortably established.

During later childhood play remains important but can be more direct. Children are often interested in using their developing learning and thinking skills to show what they can do and to enter into the activities around them.

Adolescents often need peers in order to relate to any adult. When someone their own age is present, interactions are more relaxed and spontaneous. Once they begin to know an adult in the presence of peers, establishing individual contact becomes more comfortable.

Behavior guidance and counseling

One of the most consistent concerns of parents is the adequacy, acceptability, and appropriateness of their child's behavior. In many instances their concern is so intense that they seek counsel from anyone who is even vaguely concerned with their child. Therefore, the health care worker is often asked to provide guidance for parents who desire assistance with the rearing of their child.

The goal of the family unit is to rear children who, as individuals, can accept themselves and control their behavior to an extent that is acceptable to others and who can move from the family unit with ease. Generally, conflicts are minimal in the family where individuality is rewarded, fostered, and respected. This type of family tends to facilitate the development of a personal sense of identity that is strong and not subject to serious conflicts later in life. Children need freedom to experience a wide variety of behaviors in finding their own identity, but they also need culturally acceptable guidelines for behavior. Often children are uncomfortable because they lack clear parental guidance to develop a set of norms for themselves. In recent societies peers have become important sources of behavioral norms, since there are few traditional restrictions placed on behavior by the family. Primary areas in which parents continue to provide limits include assurance of safety, respect for the rights of others, respect for property, and respect for the quality of the physical and psychologic environments.

It should be understood that there are no set universal standards of normal behavior. Adequate behavior is environmentally and culturally determined. One family may consciously or unconsciously foster behavior in a child that another family finds unacceptable. Some parents believe it is important that their children be raised within the norms by which they as children were raised. Other parents seek to rear their children according to the mode of the latest popular book on the subject. Often there is a struggle within the parent between an alliance to an inherited cultural standard and a desire to provide a more self-directed child-rearing approach. Many parents are additionally perplexed by the wide range of behavior that is tolerable, especially in recent societies, where the environment is a composite of many cultural influences. It is not uncommon, for instance, for a parent to be concerned with "what the neighbors might think." This is an unpredictable and frustrating concern for both the parent and the child in the transient and culturally disperse climate that presently exists.

Not only is behavior environmentally and culturally determined, but it is also determined by the capacity of the child. Novice parents may have heard about "ages and stages," but they often hold unrealistic expectations for their young child's behavior that are inconsistent with his developmental capacity. A young child who "gets into everything" may be exhibiting the normal exploration of taste, feel, touch, and smell. Only if the behavior persists into later childhood is it possibly indicative of a problem that requires professional evaluation and therapy.

Values develop in stages that parallel physical and cognitive capacities. Children at the age of 4 may feel that because they want something, they should have it. Therefore, it is acceptable, from their point of view, to take whatever they want. From the parent's point of view, this behavior may be known as stealing and should be punished. By understanding the child's developmental capacity, behavior can be dealt with in such a way that society's expectations for the respect of others' rights and property are met and yet expectations for the child's

perception and behavior are not unreasonable.

Often parents seek a professional relationship that will facilitate their own understanding of the child's behavior or that will bring about a change in undesirable behavior. When there is an expressed concern over behavior and discipline, the needs of the parents must be appropriately determined. They may need help in viewing each child as an individual and in accepting as normal their child's spontaneous behavior. Specific resources may be used that help in understanding the limitations placed on the child by the particular developmental stage, such as the information contained in Chapters 2 and 3.

In some instances a particular specialist may be needed to evaluate a problem and to establish the need for specific therapy. There are many instances, however, when parents need temporary assistance from health care workers in establishing and continuing satisfying family relationships. A few general principles that tend to facilitate such helping relationships with parents are reviewed below.

Cultural and environmental influences should be considered in determining what is expected for a particular family. The personal cultural bias of the helping person should not interfere with the parent-child relationship or with the expectations set for that relationship unless there is an obvious need for protection of the child's well-being.

The helping person should establish a goal for the relationship that is congruent with the goals of the family. Behavior change may be desirable, or there may be a more basic need for a helper who can provide empathic support during a time of crisis when change is neither possible nor desirable. The goals of the parents should be identified as clearly as possible, because these may not be accurately represented by the health care worker's perception of what is desirable. For example, a single parent who has sole responsibility for the discipline of a child may desire more effective behavior control for the child but may be fearful that the imposition of controls will foster resentment in the parent-child relationship. The health care worker may perceive the situation as the case of a "spoiled" child whose parent is unwilling to apply appropriate discipline. In reality, this parent may need only a minimal amount of support, encouragement, and reinforcement concerning a desired and valuable set of limits. A brief supportive contact in which the actual perspective is recognized may be sufficient to bring about a favorable climate in the home and help reduce tension in the child.

Observation is an important tool in identifying the nature of a problem, in determining the need for change, and in facilitating needed change. Each of the environmental and cultural resources of the family needs to be identified as it relates to the child's behavior. Identification of the factors that reinforce or cause behaviors to persist may require specialized skill and experience in working with particular behavioral problems. However, it may be possible for the general health care worker or the parents themselves to identify relevant circumstances that need to be changed in order to bring about positive change in the child's behavior. The techniques of behavior modification or other forms of behavior therapy can be enlisted by skilled practitioners when a problem persists despite the problem-solving efforts of the parents and the health care worker.

The nature of the parent-child relationship may yield useful clues in regard to the child's behavior. The kind of eye contact, physical touch, verbal tones, and disciplinary messages that are used in parent-child communication can help to identify the parent's resources in attempting to rear the child. The parent's perception of the child is often readily communicated through verbal and nonverbal messages both to the child and to professional helpers. Parents give clues as to whether they have a low regard or an adoring attitude toward the child. They may indicate that they view the child as a burden or that they enjoy the child. They give indications of the level of expectations for the child's behavior and of conditions that must be met in order for the child to win their love and affection. It is often observed that parental perceptions of the child and his or her behavior are fulfilled. The child who is viewed as an inadequate, unattractive, burdensome individual will reflect these traits in behavior and in self-esteem. The child who is placed under stringent conditions in order to win the love and affection of the parents is tense and overacts to meet the conditions set.

Unfortunately there are parents who have extremely limited resources in child-rearing. They are not equipped either personally, culturally, or economically to deal with the responsibilities of a child. Poverty, unhappy adult and marriage relationships, overbearing and manipulative relatives, illness, and other forms of family stress can leave a parent inadequate to respond to the needs of the child. In addition, occasionally there is a parent who cannot accept the parent role or who rejects a particular child within the family unit. When such circumstances exist, the welfare of the child becomes a primary concern, and the best possible conditions for the health and well-being of the child must be established. Long-term professional counseling may be necessary for some families, or the child may need to be placed outside of the primary family unit for a period of time.

Behavioral guidance depends on the nature of the environment, norms of the culture, expectations of the family, and the physical, developmental, and mental stage or capacity of the child. The appropriate strategy for providing parental guidance is established by attending to communication and observing interactions within the family unit and other features of the child's environment. When the problem is perceived to be beyond the capability of the health care worker, appropriate consultation should be obtained.

THE PROBLEM-ORIENTED RECORD

Each component of the problem-oriented record is described briefly as follows.

The *data base* is the initial evaluation of the child. The information to be included in the data base is defined in advance for all children seen by a given practitioner or in a given situation. The assessment tools in Chapter 10 provide examples of a complete data base for children.

The *health status list* (problem list) is extracted from the information obtained in the data base. The more adequate the data base, the more accurate the health status list will be. This list is entered at the front of the patient's chart and is permanent. Each problem is numbered consecutively as it is entered, and the list becomes an index to the entire record, since progress notes are made relative to each problem by number. All known problems are listed, including physiologic, psychologic, and socioeconomic problems. A health need or problem title is not listed as a diagnosis unless it can be unquestionably confirmed by the data. Titles begin as subjective symptoms (such as blurred vision) and are changed as more information becomes available (acute myopia).

Problem assessment and plan formulation are conducted for each health need or problem identified separately. This may be part of the initial assessment or, as new problems arise, this description and evaluation process is employed. Within the body of the chart the problem is referred to by number and title, and the following information is then recorded:

1. *Subjective data* (S). The problem from the mother or child's point of view. Often a direct quote from the informant is given to convey more completely the person's own perception of the problem.
2. *Objective data* (O). The direct physical observation, laboratory findings, or behavioral observations that are pertinent to the present problem.
3. *Assessment* (A). The criteria that can be identified in delineating the problem. It may not be possible to make a diagnosis, but a summary statement of the subjective and objective findings can be made that reflects possible diagnostic criteria.
4. *Plan* (P). Plans for further diagnostic tests; referrals; any methods of obtaining further information; plans for therapy, for patient education, or for follow-up. Subsequent implementation of the plan may be conducted in an organized, purposeful, and efficient manner.

Progress notes and related data are entered by all members of the health care team in continuing sequence. They are made according to the format of the problem assessment and plan formulation in relation to each existing or new problem that is identified. A flow sheet may be developed for recording frequently obtained data for a specific problem. For example, if a child is being seen at frequent intervals because of a nephrotic syndrome, all of the data to be obtained at each visit, such as urinalysis results, blood pressure, and observations of physical features, might be entered on a flow sheet to facilitate comparison from one visit to another. However, the numbering system for each problem allows one to quickly identify and compare all data obtained in relation to a single problem over a period of time. In addition, health care over an extended period of time can be critically evaluated, and learning from past experience is maximized for the practitioner.

Examples of such a record may be found in each unit of *Child Health Maintenance: Concepts in Family-Centered Care.**

INTRODUCTION TO THE ASSESSMENT

The health history, assessment, and subsequent plan for action can be conceptualized as aiming toward fulfillment of four major competencies throughout the developmental period.

1. *Physical competency.* This includes the child's ability to use various motor and neurologic capacities to attain mobility and manipulation capabilities and to physically take care of biologic and physiologic needs. Children begin totally helpless and immobile and grow gradually to the point where they are able to maintain physical health and provide for physical performance and mobility.

2. *Learning and thought competency.* This includes the development of language and thought processes, cognitive maps and abstractions, perception, and communication capabilities. At birth children are able to crudely communicate a few basic physiologic needs, and they begin to assimilate multiple stimuli, which eventually grow into conceptualizations and cognitive structures.

3. *Social competency.* This includes the child's development of interpersonal relationships, including affiliations with significant adults and peers, and sociocultural interactions

---

*Chinn, P. L.: St. Louis, 1979, The C. V. Mosby Co.

with individuals and groups of people. The processes of separation and affiliation constantly interact until the individual is able, during adulthood, to attain security and comfort from a variety of interpersonal relationships.

4. *Inner competency.* This includes the individual's developing awareness of self and the ability to cope as a separate person with the multitude of factors that influence the self. The child at first experiences self as a part of others and is not able to assume responsibility and accountability for his or her own thoughts, behavior, or being until maturity is achieved. An inner sense of security and well-being characterizes the healthy child at any stage of development. The development of personality traits that are characteristic for each stage of life has been identified through the various theories of personality development.

These four major competencies develop simultaneously and constantly interact and influence one another. They may be enhanced or caused to deteriorate by the multiple factors influencing development, and in fact each competency becomes a factor influencing the others.

History

The history must contain certain specific information that is suggested in the outline in Chapter 2. This is elicited through appropriate interpersonal interactions with the parent and with the child. One observation period of child-parent relationships may give a grossly inaccurate picture. If there is any question as to the adequacy of the child's interactions, past developmental course, or environmental condition, a home visit to further substantiate the impressions of inadequacy may be initiated. It should be remembered that the observer's presence will detract somewhat from the validity of the observations. In order to gain a feeling for the adequacy of the child's total environment, the child may be asked directly such questions as "Are you happy?" "Do you have friends?" "What do you like best to do?" "Do you hurt anywhere?" "Is anything making you sad?" The health worker is concerned not only with children's physical and developmental processes but also with how they feel about

themselves and how they view the world around them.

Physical assessment

Physical assessment of the child proceeds somewhat differently from assessment of the adult. The health worker must become skilled in judging the appropriate moment to proceed with certain portions of the examination. Few child assessments follow a predictable pattern or structure. Although the assessment is ordered in this guide generally from head to toe (see Chapter 2), an entirely different approach may be appropriate for each child. The infant or toddler objects to having the head examined; thus this may be left until last for this age child. If the child is crying, it is not possible to palpate the abdomen effectively, but the throat might be most effectively visualized.

During examination of a child a few principles should be noted. First, the child should be kept warm. Although it is necessary to disrobe the child for portions of the examination, the child should be kept warm and protected from drafts. Second, the child's comfort and security must be considered. Frustrating delays and uncomfortable procedures should be avoided. If pain and discomfort must be inflicted for any reason, this should be approached honestly and terminated quickly, followed by appropriate comfort and sympathy. Rewarding a painful experience with treats, candy, or excessive attention is not a sound practice. Finally, the child's safety must be considered. The assumption should never be made that an infant is too young to roll off the edge of a table or that a toddler is reliable enough not to try jumping from a table. Sharp pins and objects such as scissors should be carefully guarded away from the child's reach. All medications and toxic substances stored in the clinic or the clinician's bag should be carefully protected from the reach of a child of any age.

Most of the assessment can be conducted while the infant or child is in the parent's lap or sitting on a chair. A clinic setting is often an inhibiting factor in making a reliable assessment, and every effort should be made to arrange the room in such a manner as to facilitate the comfort of the child and parent. The child's own home is often a more conducive setting for the major portion of the assessment. Forceful restraint is usually unnecessary and should be used only as a last resort. The climate of the assessment should allow for natural behavior between the parent and the child. Much of the assessment may be completed by watching the child's normal behavior and play, and the reliability of the observations is greatly increased.

The four major techniques of the physical assessment are:

1. Observation and inspection
2. Palpation (light and deep)
3. Percussion (The third finger of the right hand strikes the underlying third finger terminal phalanx of the left hand, which is placed firmly over the skin. The other fingers must be kept off the patient's skin to keep from dampening the percussion note.)
4. Auscultation (A quality pediatric stethoscope is most useful in localizing the child's heart and breath sounds.)

Basic equipment used in the assessment includes:

1. Stethoscope
2. Blood pressure apparatus with a variety of cuff sizes
3. Thermometer
4. Pocket flashlight
5. Tongue blade
6. Reflex hammer
7. Tuning fork
8. Ophthalmoscope with otoscope
9. Tape measure

Facilities for obtaining hemoglobin or hematocrit measures, urinalysis, throat culture, vision screening, Denver Developmental Screening Test, and reliable weighing should be available in a clinic. Toys, books, and simple play equipment should always be available for use in approaching the child, in helping the child to achieve comfort in the health care setting, and in developmental assessment and observation.

CHAPTER 2

Assessment of physical competency

OUTLINE OF THE HISTORY, ENVIRONMENTAL INTERVIEW, AND PHYSICAL ASSESSMENT

The following outline is intended to serve several purposes. It may be used as a guide for learning and practice in attaining skill and thoroughness in health assessment of children. It may be used to determine the adequacy of the health assessment performed by students and practitioners. It may be used as a guide for recording the data base obtained in the health assessment. The user is encouraged to make adjustments, modifications, and expansions to fit the kind of practice in which he or she is engaged and to provide for individual creativity in practice.

Although this outline is intended as a guide, it should not be used as a "questionnaire" for the parent or the child. Skill should be developed in eliciting this information on an individualized basis, with primary attention to developing interpersonal relationships with the family and child.

  I. History
    A. Paternal history
      1. History of chronic illness in the father's family
      2. Previous medical-surgical events
      3. Present health status
      4. Age

    B. Maternal history
      1. History of chronic illness in the mother's family
      2. Previous medical-surgical events
      3. History of previous pregnancies
      4. Prenatal history
        a. Medical supervision
        b. Diet, nutrition
        c. Illnesses, infections, or complications
        d. Medications
        e. Treatment and procedures required
      5. Natal history for this child
        a. Duration of pregnancy
        b. Course of labor and delivery
        c. Sedation/anesthesia required
      6. Date of last menstrual period (include any needed family planning counsel)
      7. Age
    C. Child
      1. Physical competency
        a. Neonatal status
          (1) Risk classification
          (2) Apgar score
          (3) Congenital abnormalities
        b. Postnatal course
        c. Previous illnesses
        d. Accidents and injuries
        e. Medications
        f. Fluid and caloric intake or nutrition history (see p. 108)
        g. Developmental milestones (see DDST, p. 67)
        h. Growth patterns and weight changes

      i. Allergies
      j. Immunizations (see p. 82)
  2. Learning and thought competency
    a. Language development (see DDST and PRESS, pp. 67 and 79)
    b. School progress
  3. Social competency
    a. Personal social development (see DDST, p. 67)
    b. Mother-child or father-child relationship based on observation of eye contact, touching, tone of voice of parent, ease of separation, mutual free expression, mutual activities, behaviors reinforced, methods of punishment, and so on
    c. Parent substitutes
    d. Position in family
    e. Social climate in home
    f. Climate in school
  4. Inner competency
    a. Structure described in such concepts as the following (based on behavioral observations):
      (1) Rigidity-flexibility
      (2) Accuracy-inaccuracy
      (3) Simplicity-complexity
      (4) Breadth-narrowness
    b. Function
      (1) Self-evaluation and ability for introspection
      (2) Prediction of success or failure
      (3) Obtaining personal survival, acceptance, comfort, enhancement, competence, and actualization of realization
      (4) Instigation of behavior mediated by child's own desires and values or by society's desires and values
    c. Quality
      (1) High or low self-esteem
II. Environmental interview
  A. Pollutants (air, water, radiation, and so on) (see p. 85)
  B. Environmental hazards
    1. Population density
    2. Infestations (microbiologic, animal)
    3. Lead ingestion
    4. Firearms in the home
    5. Medication/poisons
    6. Disposal or collection of garbage
    7. Fire hazards
    8. Crime
    9. Transportation for medical care and emergencies

  C. Fluoridation of water supply (see p. 85)
  D. Psychologic-social environment
    1. Appearance of home and community
    2. Sound stimuli
    3. Social climate of community
    4. Psychologic and social impact of environmental hazards
    5. Life-style of family
III. Physical assessment (see Assessment guide, pp. 13-37)
  A. Body measurements
    1. Head circumference
    2. Chest circumference
    3. Height
    4. Weight
  B. Vital signs
    1. Temperature
    2. Pulse rate
    3. Respiratory rate
    4. Blood pressure
  C. Neuromuscular system
    1. Neuromuscular history
    2. Present neurologic status
      a. Social affect
      b. Developmental status
      c. Speech development
      d. Memory
      e. Posture, muscle tone
      f. Reflexes
      g. Cranial nerve function
      h. Cerebellar function
      i. Fine motor coordination
      j. Parietal lobe function
      k. Proprioception
      l. Tactile capacity
  D. Skin
    1. Condition and description
    2. Hydration
  E. Head
    1. Measurement of circumference
    2. Measurement of fontanels
    3. Transillumination
    4. Palpation
  F. Face
    1. Expression
    2. Palpebral fissures
    3. Placement of ears
    4. Percussion of sinuses
    5. Skin
  G. Hair and scalp
    1. Hairline
    2. Hygiene
  H. Eyes
    1. Visual acuity
    2. Amblyopia

3. Peripheral fields
4. Color
5. Motor function
6. Strabismus
7. Retina
8. Conjunctivae and lids
9. Vision behavior

I. Nose
   1. Patency of nostrils
   2. Discharge
   3. Olfactory sense

J. Mouth and throat
   1. Teeth and gums
   2. Pharynx
   3. Tongue
   4. Hard and soft palates
   5. Throat culture
   6. Swallowing capacity

K. Ears
   1. Structure
   2. Function of hearing

L. Neck
   1. Palpation
   2. Motion

M. Chest
   1. Axillary nodes
   2. Nipples and breast tissue

N. Heart
   1. Size and position
   2. Apex beat
   3. Description of sounds

O. Lungs
   1. Respiratory movement
   2. Description of sounds

P. Abdomen
   1. Size and contour
   2. Percussion of organs
   3. Auscultation
   4. Umbilicus
   5. Femoral pulses

Q. Back and spine
   1. Structure

R. Extremities
   1. Inspection of arms and legs
   2. Palmar creases
   3. Function and mobility of joints
   4. Hip abduction

S. Urinary system
   1. Characteristics of voiding
   2. Urinalysis

T. Genitalia
   1. Structural adequacy
   2. Secondary sexual characteristics

U. Anus
   1. Structure
   2. Function

Physical assessment guide

Procedure	Expected findings (age dependent)	Deviations	Implications for health care
	BODY MEASUREMENTS		
	See Chapter 4. All body measurements should fall within expected limits of measurement as indicated on the growth graphs in Chapter 4. The child should maintain about the same percentile ranking on each measurement throughout childhood. Percentile rankings from one area to another are usually similar for one child but may vary (for example, a child may be at the 25th percentile for height and the 10th percentile for weight).	A sudden or gradual shift in the previously established percentile for a measurement. Unusually deviant variations in percentile between areas of measurement, such as a child who is at the 25th percentile for height and the 97th percentile for weight.	Growth problems at any age require specialist evaluation.
1. HEAD CIRCUMFERENCE Measure at greatest diameter, occiput to frontal areas.	During infancy: approximates the size of the infant's chest.	Beyond limits of normal on growth graph.	Determine adequacy of all neurologic signs.
2. CHEST CIRCUMFERENCE Measure at level of the nipples after exhalation.	Lateral diameter of chest should be greater than anteroposterior diameter.	Increased circumference; barreling of chest.	Determine adequacy of other respiratory and circulatory signs.
3. HEIGHT Measure recumbent length until age 6 years; standing height after age 6 years.	Plotted within expectations as determined by growth graphs. Estimate guide: $2 \times$ age in years + 32 = approximate height in inches.	Retarded or excessive growth. Disproportionate growth compared with weight.	Determine other signs of skeletal system adequacy.
4. WEIGHT Measure body weight in light underclothing.	Plotted with expectations as determined by growth graphs. Estimate guides: 1st year of life: age in months + 11 = weight in pounds. 1st year to puberty: $5 \times$ age in years + 18 = weight in pounds.	Retarded or excessive gains in weight. Weight disproportionate to height.	Determine nutritional adequacy, genetic predisposition for body build, emotional factors of the environment. Parental guidance for appropriate caloric intake may be indicated. Specialist consultation indicated for planning and implementing caloric therapy during childhood.
	VITAL SIGNS		
1. TEMPERATURE Obtain axillary temperature with glass thermometer in those under age 6 years; oral temperature in those over age 6 years.	See Chapter 4. Normally higher than adults; axillary or oral temperature below 100.5° F is generally considered within normal limits.	Elevated above about 101° F.	See Chapter 6 (Common illnesses).

Continued.

Physical assessment guide—cont'd

Procedure	Expected findings (age dependent)	Deviations	Implications for health care
	VITAL SIGNS—cont'd		
2. PULSE RATE Obtain by auscultation of heart rate in infants and young children; determine adequacy of pulse in each extremity and femoral area.	Pulse rate is increased after exercise or crying but should return to a preexercise level within 5-10 minutes. Athletes in training may have a normally slower heart rate. Approximate rates (see p. 63): 0-12 months: 130/min. 1-2 years: 105/min. 2-5 years: 90/min. 5-12 years: 75/min. 12-18 years: 65/min.	Tachycardia. Bradycardia.	See p. 32 (Heart).
3. RESPIRATORY RATE Obtain while child is in a quiet, resting state.	Rate increases in response to exercise or crying. Approximate rates (see p. 63): 0-12 months: 30/min. 1-5 years: 26/min. 5-12 years: 20/min. 12-18 years: 18/min.	Increased or decreased rates; Cheyne-Stokes respirations.	See p. 33 (Lungs). Emergency intervention to ensure adequate gas exchange.
4. BLOOD PRESSURE Adequate cuff size is essential. The width of the cuff should slightly exceed the lateral diameter of the extremity where the cuff is to be placed.	Approximate pressures (see p. 64): Newborn: 80/46. 1 year: 96/66. 5 years: 94/55. 12 years: 114/60.	Unusual increase or decrease in pressures.	Correlate increases with protein in urine, edema, obesity, or visual disturbances. Decreases indicate immediate emergency provision for adequacy of circulation.
	NEUROMUSCULAR SYSTEM		
Determine neuromuscular developmental history.	Normal past development.	History of headaches; transient loss of consciousness; episodes of weakness, numbness in extremities, convulsions.	Indications of past signs of neuromuscular problems require specialist evaluation.
1. Determine present neurologic status. a. Appraise social affect and manner; obtain evidence of child's judgment and insight, considering cultural influences.	Apropriate for age and stage of development: To 6 or 8 months: responds to nonfamily and family members alike. Fear of strangers and separation anxiety occur at about 7 months. 2 years: plays simple interactive games. 3 years: separates from mother easily. Early childhood: parallel play predominates.	Inappropriate degrees of: Depression. Hyperactivity. Hypoactivity. Distractibility. Impulsiveness. Aloofness. Lack of social response. Deficient speech. Preoccupation with objects. Delayed social development.	Determine other neurologic signs. Indications of neurologic inadequacy require specialist evaluation. Mother and caretakers may need counseling and support with social problems or with provision of adequate stimulation.

Physical assessment guide—cont'd

Procedure	Expected findings (age dependent)	Deviations	Implications for health care
	NEUROMUSCULAR SYSTEM—cont'd		
	Later childhood: interaction with children of the same sex may predominate; peers become important in determining behavior. Adolescence: dependence on peers of both sexes predominates.	Precocious social development in combination with excessive adult contacts. Constant isolation imposed by caretakers or by the child himself. Lack of environmental stimulation. Overprotection by caretakers. Excessive identity with one person.	Culturally appropriate reading material may enhance parenting ability. Refer to mental health worker if problems interfere with child's ability to function adequately.
b. Administer available standardized tools, such as:			Use standard criteria for referral to specialists.
Denver Developmental Screening Test (DDST).	See p. 67.		
Preschool Readiness Experimental Screening Scale (PRESS).	See p. 80.		
Denver Articulation Screening Examination (DASE).	See p. 73.		
c. Appraise general speech development (see Chapter 4).	Newborn: medium-pitched cry.	High-pitched cry.	Determine other neurologic signs.
	6 months: babbles, imitates speech sounds. 18 months: uses about 10 words. 2 years: uses 2- to 3-word sentences.	Delayed speech and language development.	Determine ability to hear. Determine social adequacy of child's environment.
	3 years: able to communicate with nonfamily members effectively for basic desires.		Specific teaching regarding language stimulation and communication with child.
	6 years: complete basic grammar, 90% fluent in language of the home.		Persistent problem indicates need for education or medical specialist evaluation.

Continued.

Physical assessment guide—cont'd

Procedure	Expected findings (age dependent)	Deviations	Implications for health care
	NEUROMUSCULAR SYSTEM—cont'd		
d. Appraise memory. Under 5 years: use memory-related items on the DDST and PRESS. School-age: consult with parent or teacher.	Appropriate for age.		
e. Appraise posture and muscle tone by observing child's activities and movement characteristics.	POSTURE Infancy: Supine—may assume a tonic neck or fencing position. Prone—will turn head to one side, raise it off the table, and make creeping motions with legs; lies at rest with arms and legs drawn close to body. Sitting—sits unsupported by age 8 months.	Delayed or abnormal postural development. Asymmetry of tone or strength. Tremors. Abnormal flexions or extensions.	Counseling with mother regarding developmental milestones for individual child; need for spatial and kinesthetic exploration and for safety provisions as mobility increases. Delays indicate need for specialist evaluation.
	Early childhood: Standing posture is characterized by swaying of spine (toddler lordosis). This disappears by age 3½-4 years. Walking alone by age 18 months with spine straight. Hips move symmetrically, with knees straight and feet maintained in straight alignment.	"Knock knees." "Flat feet" accompanied by aching feet or legs that tire with exercise. "Pidgeon toes." Opisthotonos (pitched frog position). Hemiparesis (may be accompanied by clenching of the fist on the affected side).	Counseling with mother regarding symptoms of concern, including discussion of "normal" and "abnormal" alignment. Referral to a specialist is required if persistent clumsiness or discomfort is associated. May imply neuromuscular condition that needs referral to specialist immediately.
	Later childhood: when child bends over to touch his toes, spine moves in straight alignment, with symmetrical curve to shoulders and hips.	Asymmetry of curve of spine, level of shoulders, or hips.	Indicates need for orthopedic evaluation and treatment.
	Adolescence: may exhibit postural inadequacies related to peak growth acceleration. Adult postural characteristics should be established within several months of this change.	Inadequacies of skeletal growth during adolescence.	Indicates need for specialist evaluation.

Physical assessment guide—cont'd

Procedure	Expected findings (age dependent)	Deviations	Implications for health care
	NEUROMUSCULAR SYSTEM—cont'd		
	MUSCLE TONE AND MOVEMENT CHARACTERISTICS		
	Newborn:	Delayed or abnormal development.	Anticipatory guidance for advancing muscle and strength capacities.
	Symmetrical strength in all extremities. Movement may be jerky. Head lag not over 45°.	Asymmetry of tone or strength.	
	Neck control should be present to maintain head erect briefly.	Tremors.	
	Child: symmetry of movement; adequate gross and fine motor development.	Asymmetry; tremors; delayed ability to perform fine and gross motor tasks.	Evaluate adequacy of environmental opportunities for stimulation and motor exercise.
			Persistent inadequacies indicate the need for specialist evaluation.
2. Test reflexes to determine meningeal irritability.			These three signs are symptomatic of meningeal irritation and indicate need for immediate medical care.
a. Paradoxical irritability.	Child is calmed with physical cuddling and rocking (given that he is not hungry, frightened, or in pain).	Child cries when held (paradoxical irritability).	
b. Kernig's sign: bend the thigh at the hip and attempt to extend the leg at the knee.	Leg is extended easily and without pain.	Extension of the leg at the knee gives pain and resistance (Kernig's sign).	
c. Brudzinski's sign: bend the neck while child is supine and note flexion of the knees.	No movement is noted in the legs when the neck is flexed.	Knees bend spontaneously with passive flexion of the neck (Brudzinski's sign).	
3. Test infant reflexes.			
a. Moro reflex: allow head and trunk to fall backward from a sitting position through an angle of at least 30°.	Symmetrical extension and abduction of arms with fingers extended and fanned, thumb and index finger forming a "C" shape. There may be a slight tremor, then a return to relaxed flexion and/or normal movement.	Asymmetry of response suggests injury or paralysis.	Teaching of parents who are not familiar with this response may allay worry when it is observed to occur at home in response to sudden movement or loud noises.
	Birth-8 weeks: present.		
	8-18 weeks: body jerk only.		
	6 months: should be absent.	Absent reflex indicates severe neurologic deficit before 8 weeks of age.	Specialist evaluation indicated.

Continued.

Physical assessment guide—cont'd

Procedure	Expected findings (age dependent)	Deviations	Implications for health care
NEUROMUSCULAR SYSTEM—cont'd			
b. Sucking and rooting reflexes: observe infant during feeding.	Roots toward tactile stimulus on cheeks, grasps nipple firmly, and sucks spontaneously. Sucking lasts sufficiently to take adequate feedings. Responses absent if infant has just been fed.	Absence of responses indicates low gestational age or neurologic damage. Exhaustibility of responses may indicate low gestational age.	Feeding assistance and teaching may be indicated for mother. Determine adequacy of weight gain if inadequacies of sucking are detected.
c. Palmar and plantar grasps: place finger in palm of hands and at base of toes.	Palmar: fingers grasp examiner's finger. Response lessens by 3-4 months. Plantar: toes curl downward. Response lessens by 8 months.	Asymmetry of responses.	Determine other infantile reflexes.
d. Babinski reflex: stroke one side of sole of foot upward and across ball of foot.	Infant: hyperextension of all toes. Child: flexion of all toes.	Infant: absence of response. Child: hyperextension of all toes or absence of response.	Abnormal findings indicate need for specialist evaluation.
e. Stepping: support infant vertically above table and place one foot in contact with surface.	Normal infant will step alternately.	Asymmetry of stepping.	Determine use and muscle tone on each side of body; may need specialist evaluation.
f. Landau reflex: suspend infant in prone position over table.	When suspended in prone position, infant tends to maintain spine in a horizontal position with the head above horizontal plane by 3 months of age. By 10 months, spine is slightly concave and head is lifted above horizontal plane.	Absence of postural responses to the position.	
g. Incurvation of the trunk: with infant lying prone on the table, run finger down paravertebral area on both sides of the spine.	1-4 weeks: swinging of pelvis toward the stimulated side. Response disappears after 4 weeks of age.		
h. Tonic neck reflex: turn head sharply to one side.	Ipsilateral arm and leg extend and opposite ones flex in a fencing position. Response disappears by 3-4 months.	This response may not be observed and is not considered a reliable indication of neurologic function.	All neurologic deficits indicate a need for specialist evaluation.

Physical assessment guide—cont'd

Procedure	Expected findings (age dependent)	Deviations	Implications for health care
	NEUROMUSCULAR SYSTEM—cont'd		
4. Test childhood and adolescent reflexes. a. Babinski.	See above.		
b. Strike reflex hammer to biceps, triceps, and brachioradialis.	Symmetry of response in both arms.	Hyperreflexia. Reflexes missing or weak after repeated trials.	
c. Strike reflex hammer to knee (patellar), Achilles tendon.	Symmetry of response in both knees and feet.	Asymmetry of response. Hyperreflexia. Reflexes missing or weak.	Evaluate in the light of other neurologic findings.
5. Test eye reflexes. See p. 75 (Vision).			
6. Test cranial nerve function. I (olfactory) II (optic) III, IV, and VI (oculomotor, trochlear, and abducens) V (trigeminal) VII (facial) VIII (acoustic) IX, X (glossopharyngeal and vagus) XI (accessory) XII (hypoglossal)	See p. 26. See p. 24. See p. 25. See p. 23. See p. 23. See p. 28. See p. 28. See p. 31. See p. 27.		
7. Test cerebellar function. a. Appraise large motor coordination by having the child do the following:	Range of coordination or clumsiness is considerable. Most children can perform these tasks by age 3 years; coordination and skill increase with age.	Obvious incoordination, with inability to perform on one side particularly. Incoordination and loss of function that was previously present.	A young child who has lacked environmental opportunities to perform these tasks will appear deficient in function. Environmental stimulation may be applied for a period of time and re-evaluation made after several weeks.
Run in place.	Runs with equal gait, is able to maintain balance, coordinates arm and leg movements effectively.	Exaggerated motions, inability to maintain balance and equal gait.	
Balance on one foot with eyes closed (Rhomberg test).	Able to balance for several seconds.	Unable to achieve balance with eyes closed.	Obvious inabilities, incoordination, or other deficiencies require specialist evaluation.
Walk heel-to-toe.	Able to walk for several steps without losing balance; uses arms effectively in maintaining balance.	Unable to perform without losing balance.	

Continued.

Physical assessment guide—cont'd

Procedure	Expected findings (age dependent)	Deviations	Implications for health care
	NEUROMUSCULAR SYSTEM—cont'd		
Touch tip of nose with index finger with eyes closed.	Able to bring finger to nose without groping or tremors.	Gropes for nose-finger contact, touches the side or bridge of nose, and cannot bring finger to tip of nose.	
Copy the following hand movements:			
Tap hands back and forth on top of examiner's hands.	Able to alternate tapping palm and back of hands.	Unable to make alternating motion.	
Pat each thigh with palms, doing both at the same time.	Able to tap hands simultaneously, maintaining even rhythm.	Unable to coordinate movements of each hand together or to maintain rhythm.	
Twist both hands as though screwing a light bulb.	Able to copy twisting motion in both hands.	Unable to copy twisting motion to either hand.	
b. Appraise fine motor coordination as follows:			
Infant: observe pincer grasp.	Appears by 9-12 months.		
Child: observe ability to draw and to copy geometric shapes.	18 months: scribbles spontaneously. 2½-4 years: copies geometric shapes. 10 years: able to control execution of lines to achieve desired effect.	Obvious incoordination. Inability to perform when previous ability was present. Developmental delay (see DDST, p. 67).	Child who has lacked environmental opportunity to perform these tasks will appear deficient in function. Environmental stimulation may be appropriate. Obvious inabilities, incoordination, or other deficiencies require specialist evaluation. Behavioral evidence of child's appropriate abilities may be useful in counseling and guidance for family in understanding normal development.

Physical assessment guide—cont'd

Procedure	Expected findings (age dependent)	Deviations	Implications for health care
NEUROMUSCULAR SYSTEM—cont'd			
8. Test parietal lobe function.			
a. Have child put right thumb on left eye.	Knows right from left by age 7-9 years.		
b. Have child close eyes; put a small object in child's hand and ask him or her to identify it.	Able to identify most common objects, such as coins, keys, buttons, paper clips, rubber bands.	Inability to perform tasks and identify small objects.	May have lacked environmental opportunities to develop skills and knowledge. Stimulation may be appropriate.
9. Test proprioception. Have child close eyes; move toe in either an upward/downward or backward/forward motion.	Child is able to identify the direction of the movement.	Unable to detect the direction of movement.	Evaluate in light of other neurologic findings.
10. Test tactile capacity. Have child close eyes. Touch areas of child's body and extremities with a cold object such as a tuning fork.	Child is able to identify the location of the sensation in all areas.	Does not feel the sensory stimuli.	Evaluate in light of other neurologic findings.
SKIN			
1. Inspect the skin and make a thorough description of unusual conditions.	Color normal for ethnic group. Birthmarks. Moles. Scars. Minor bruises. Mongolian spots on infant's buttocks.	Rashes. Open lesions. Any mole or growth that changes in size, color, character. Multiple bruises, scars, especially if associated with limited range of motion and soreness.	Mild, nonspecific rashes: instruct mother in adequate care of skin with minimal use of cleansing agents, which might be irritating. (See p. 95 for diaper rash.) Treat allergies, infections, impetigo, insect bites, specific rashes, and so on per MP* (see pp. 95-97). Identify possibility of battering; social and community mental health referral may be indicated.

*Management protocol.

Continued.

Physical assessment guide—cont'd

Procedure	Expected findings (age dependent)	Deviations	Implications for health care

SKIN—cont'd

Procedure	Expected findings (age dependent)	Deviations	Implications for health care
2. Observe skin turgor and state of hydration.	Skin elastic; pinched skin returns to normal configuration when released.	Dehydration: Dry skin. Parched tongue. Sunken fontanel. Decreased urinary output. Irritability. Lethargy. Specific gravity of urine greater than 1.030. Recent weight loss of over 6% of body weight.	Teaching regarding adequate hydration and emergency treatment. Identify source of water loss. Institute adequate fluid intake immediately. Refer for hospitalization if loss is severe (see p. 86).
		Overhydration: Diuresis. Weakness, lethargy. Drowsiness. Ileus, vomiting. Edema, weight gain. Decreased specific gravity of urine. Coma and delirium. Convulsions.	Determine adequacy of renal function and cardiovascular or respiratory involvement. Refer for hospitalization if severe.

HEAD

Procedure	Expected findings (age dependent)	Deviations	Implications for health care
1. Measure circumference (see pp. 61-62).	See growth graphs (Chapter 4).	Inadequate, excessive, or asymmetrical growth.	Mother may need instructions to rotate infant's head while sleeping to maintain symmetrical shape. If asymmetry persists, specialist evaluation is needed.
2. Measure fontanels.	Anterior: 4-6 cm in each dimension at birth. Closes by 18 months of age. Posterior: 0.5-1 cm at birth. Closes by 2 months of age. Fontanels may bulge with crying; pulse is palpable at anterior fontanel.	Sunken with dehydration. Bulging with increased intracranial pressure. Increases rather than decreases in dimensions over the period of infancy.	Correct hydration problems (see p. 93). Specialist evaluation is required for signs of increased intracranial pressure.
3. Transilluminate head (infant).	Less than 1 cm transillumination around cone on frontal area; decreases to minimal or none at base of occiput.	Excessive transillumination in any hemisphere.	Neurologic referral.
4. Palpate head for nodes and for subcutaneous or subdural swelling.	Infant: cephalhematoma may persist to 3 months. Caput succedaneum disappears by 1 week. Child: intermittent movable nodes may be detected.	Nonmovable nodes Dramatic growth in node size.	Support and reassurance for parents regarding these problems. Specialist referral.

Physical assessment guide—cont'd

Procedure	Expected findings (age dependent)	Deviations	Implications for health care
Face			
1. Appraise facial expression, alertness, interest, emotions, response to others.	Symmetry of facial expression. Interest, alertness, and expression responses appropriate for age.	Abnormal facies may occur with chromosomal syndromes such as Down's syndrome, cretinism, gargoylism. Inequality may be due to minor injury at birth and may be transient.	Specialist evaluation for diagnosis and treatment. Counseling and support of parents.
2. Appraise equality of palpebral fissures.	Equal.	Inequality may signal permanent disability.	
3. Observe relationship of ears to outer canthus of eye.	Even on a horizontal plane.	Low-set ears may be associated with renal problems or other congenital anomalies.	Specialist evaluation indicated.
4. Percuss over facial sinuses of older child and adolescent.	Should be resonant, painless.	Nonresonant, painful.	Antihistamines per MP if evidence of allergy is present. Repeated attacks or presence of specific related symptoms require specialist evaluation.
5. Appraise skin on face.	Milia may be present across nose and forehead; usually disappears by 6 weeks of age. Diffuse maculopapular rash may be present, especially in heat.	See Skin, p. 21.	Reassurance for parents regarding bothersome appearance of infant's face.
6. Assess function of trigeminal nerve (V). Sensory: test ability of child to detect light touch in maxillary and mandibular areas; test corneal reflex by touching cornea lightly and observing blink reflex.	Able to detect light touch in all facial areas; blinks in response to corneal touch. Responses equal on both sides of face.	Absence of response. Inequality of response.	Evaluate in light of other neurologic findings.
Motor: have child bite down hard and then open jaw.	Equality of bite, coordinated jaw movement.	Inequality of bite. Incoordinated movement.	
7. Assess function of facial nerve (VII). Observe lines and contours in face. Make faces for the child to mimic, such as eye squinting, frowning, nose wrinkling.	Equality of muscle function on each side of the face.	Inequality of function.	

Continued.

Physical assessment guide—cont'd

Procedure	Expected findings (age dependent)	Deviations	Implications for health care
	Face—cont'd		
8. Assess ability to discriminate tastes of salt and sugar on the anterior portion of the tongue.	Ability to discriminate tastes.	Inability to discriminate tastes.	Evaluate environmental taste stimulation opportunities. Assess in light of other neurologic findings.
	Hair and scalp		
1. Appraise hairline and distribution of hair.	Hair evenly distributed, grows toward neck and face at edges except for "cowlicks."	Uneven distribution of hair. Hair growing toward crown may accompany chromosomal disorders.	May indicate specialist referral.
2. Appraise hygiene.	Scalp free from lesions or crusty material. Hygiene adequate.	Cradle cap in infancy. Dandruff. Lice. Complaints of persistent itchiness.	Teaching regarding routine care of hair and scalp. Treat per MP*; see p. 95. May require specialist evaluation.
	Eyes		
1. Appraise function of optic nerve (II) by screening for visual function as follows:	Age-appropriate visual development (see p. 75).		Teaching and guidance related to eye safety. Maintaining good function; eye care for prevention of illness and during emergencies.
a. Denver Eye Screening Test (DEST) for infants and preschoolers.	See p. 76.		
b. Screen for amblyopia by attracting child's attention with an object and observing reactions as each eye is covered alternately.	Continues to observe object adequately with one eye covered.	Objects to having one eye covered.	Indicates need for ophthalmologic evaluation.
c. Snellen screening for visual acuity.	See p. 77.		
d. Determine peripheral vision: wiggle finger in four fields approaching a 90° angle from behind, with child maintaining gaze straight ahead.	Detects movement at 90° angle.	Inability to detect movement until finger approaches direct line of vision.	Indicates need for ophthalmologic evaluation.

*Management protocol.

Physical assessment guide—cont'd

Procedure	Expected findings (age dependent)	Deviations	Implications for health care
	Eyes—cont'd		
e. Determine ability to see colors by using the Ishihara test if possible; otherwise elicit verbal responses to color stimuli.	Able to distinguish between colors and to give the names of colors that are known. Knowledge of colors should be present by age 4 years with appropriate environmental stimulation.	Color blindness.	Refer to educational specialist for consultation and special education assistance as indicated.
2. Appraise function of the oculomotor (III), trochlear (IV), and abducens (VI) nerves.			
a. Hold child's chin steady and have him or her follow examiner's finger moving through all hemispheres, then converging on nose.	Ability to follow movement, with coordination in each eye. Eyes maintain contact during convergence, causing the appearance of crossing of the eyes.	Incoordination in one or both eyes. Inability to maintain visual contact with moving finger. Inability to converge.	Problems indicate a need for ophthalmologic evaluation.
b. Observe function of the lids and blinking.	No ptosis. Symmetrical blink.	Ptosis. Asymmetrical blink.	
c. Screen for strabismus: shine light into eyes from 2- to 3-foot distance.	Light reflects back from center of pupil in each eye. In addition, pupils react equally, and blink reflex is present. Pupils may be observed to rapidly oscillate between constriction and dilation for a few seconds (hippus).	Strabismus present if light reflection deviates from the center of one pupil. Delayed pupil reaction to light. Asymmetrical blink.	Strabismus requires immediate ophthalmologic diagnosis and treatment. Evaluate in light of other neurologic signs. Probably indicates needs for emergency specialist intervention.
3. Appraise structure of the eyes.			
a. Red reflex: shine ophthalmoscope on zero lens on pupil from a distance of 2 to 3 feet.	Red reflex from retina. 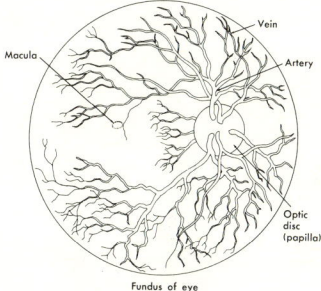 Vein Macula Artery Optic disc (papilla) Fundus of eye	Opacity of the lens.	Ophthalmologic evaluation necessary.

Continued.

Physical assessment guide—cont'd

Procedure	Expected findings (age dependent)	Deviations	Implications for health care
Eyes—cont'd			
b. Examine the retina by asking the child to focus on a spot on the wall in a darkened room. Move in the visualization of the eyegrounds, focusing with the ophthalmoscope lens.	Identify landmarks as above in each eye. The optic disc is generally pale in infancy. Pulsations can be seen through arteries.	Pallor of the disc. Edema. Suppression of pulsations. Retinal hemorrhage.	Problems indicate need for ophthalmologic evaluation.
4. Inspect conjunctivae and lids.	Moist conjunctivae and lids with dark pink color. Lids symmetrical.	Discharge, swelling, or redness indicative of infection. Ptosis. "Sty" (painful pustule on lid margin). Paleness suggestive of inadequate hemoglobin level.	Determine systemic or localized infection. Problems require specialist evaluation and treatment; MP's may be formulated for commonly observed minor eye infections and sties. Obtain hemoglobin (see Chapter 4).
5. Observe spontaneous behavior associated with visual function.	Child blinks normally at least once every 10 seconds. Reads with comfort with book about 12 inches from eyes.	Squinting. Exaggerated movements. Must hold reading material and/or head in unusual position.	Teaching and guidance related to adequate study habits and other visually related tasks. Problems may require specialist evaluation.
Nose			
1. Inspect nares. Determine patency of each nostril by obstructing flow of air in opposite nostril and mouth and observing air flow.	Patent.	Obstruction of air flow due to congenital lesion, accidental deviation of septum, foreign body, excessive secretions, irritated mucosa.	Determine source of obstruction. Remove obstruction or make appropriate referral for evaluation and correction of problem.
2. Note presence of discharge or infected lesions.	None present.	Rhinitis (allergic or infectious).	Determine source of problems. Institute therapy per MP or make appropriate referral (see Chapter 6).
3. Appraise function of olfactory nerve (I). Have child close eyes and identify odor stimuli such as chocolate, alcohol, or peanut butter.	Able to identify odor.	Unable to identify any odors.	Evaluate in light of other neurologic findings and possible presence of obstruction as above.

Physical assessment guide—cont'd

Procedure	Expected findings (age dependent)	Deviations	Implications for health care
Mouth and throat			
1. Observe condition of the teeth, gums, tongue, buccal membranes, and pharynx using adequate direct lighting and tongue blade.	Age-appropriate dental development (see p. 83).	Developmental delay.	Teaching and guidance related to oral hygiene, dental care, and treatment of minor infections and more serious illness.
	No visible dental caries. Dark pink, firm gums. Noncoated tongue.	Dental caries. Inflamed gums. Coated tongue.	Referral to dentist.
	Pharynx unobstructed, no drainage in back of throat, no exudate on tonsils.	Tonsils inflamed and enlarged to the point of obstructing the view of pharynx; exudate present.	Obtain throat culture (see Chapter 6). Determine other signs of respiratory or gastrointestinal illness.
	Tonsils may appear large and remain noninflammatory.	Strong, disagreeable odor.	
	Epstein's pearls may appear on the gums of infants.	Koplik's spots of measles.	
	Occlusion of upper and lower teeth is adequate.	Inadequate bite.	Requires orthodontic evaluation and treatment.
2. Appraise function of hypoglossal nerve (XII) by asking child to stick out the tongue and move it from side to side. Strength is determined by feeling pressure of tongue against each cheek.	Symmetry of movement and strength.	Asymmetry.	Evaluate in light of other neurologic findings.
3. Appraise intactness of newborn palate through both palpation and visualization of the entire palate.	Hard and soft palate intact.	Clefts in either hard or soft palate.	Referral to specialist is indicated.
4. Obtain culture of pharynx for group A beta hemolytic streptococci as follows: a. Illuminate throat well. b. Using sterile applicator, swab over both tonsillar areas and then over the back of the throat.	Negative for group A beta hemolytic streptococci (see Chapter 4). Gag reflex intact.	Positive culture results. Infection may be present without symptoms; thus routine throat culturing is recommended in geographic areas of risk and during seasons of highest incidence; culturing provides the only means of definitive diagnosis of this condition.	Treat per MP (see Chapter 6).

Continued.

Physical assessment guide—cont'd

Procedure	Expected findings (age dependent)	Deviations	Implications for health care
Mouth and throat—cont'd			
5. Appraise function of glossopharyngeal (IX) and vagus (X) nerves.			
a. Observe salivation.	Adequate function of mouth and pharynx.	Abnormal phonation. Suppressed reflexes. Deviations of the tongue.	Evaluate in light of other neurologic findings.
b. Observe ability to form speech sounds with the pharynx, larynx, and soft palate.			
c. Observe presence of gag reflex.			
d. Observe swallow.			
e. Observe tongue in midline.			
Ears			
1. Inspect structure of ears using otoscope; observe condition of outer ear, canal, and tympanic membrane.	External ear: flesh color accentuated with ruddiness on lobes; adequate position.	Malformation or low placement of ear. Paleness suggestive of inadequate hemoglobin level (see Chapter 4).	Determine signs of other congenital anomalies, particularly renal.
	Canal: no discharge; wax usually present in moderate amounts; no lesions; no foreign bodies.	Wax obstructing ability to hear. Discharge. Disagreeable odor. Lesions. Foreign body.	Remove wax with wire loop or curette under constant visualization.
	Tympanic membrane: gray, opaque appearance; light cone present; body landmarks present. Stapes, Handle of malleus, Umbo, Light reflex, Tympanic membrane	Redness, induration of the membrane. Absence or diffusion of the light reflex. Absence of bony landmarks.	Treat per MP (see p. 93). Repeated attacks require specialist evaluation and treatment.
2. Appraise hearing function (acoustic nerve, VIII).			
a. Newborn: determine risk of potential or existing hearing loss by determining the following:	Absence of all risk factors.	Presence of one or more risk factors.	Refer all children who have a risk factor for complete audiometric evaluation.

Physical assessment guide—cont'd

Procedure	Expected findings (age dependent)	Deviations	Implications for health care
	Ears—cont'd		
History of deafness in the family. Prematurity or low birth weight. Prolonged hospitalization at birth. Bilirubin greater than 20 during the first week of life. Malformed ears. Cleft lip or palate. Abnormal vestibular function determined by holding newborn at a 30° angle and rotating him or her in a complete circle in each direction, observing the reaction of the eyes.	Nystagmic oscillations of the eyes in the direction of the rotation.	No response.	
b. 4-18 months: test hearing response in a quiet room with child on mother's lap as follows: Distract child visually with a silent toy. Make a sound with a bell or squeeze toy close to the floor out of peripheral vision. Observe response. Repeat on opposite side.	4 months: Widening of the eyes. Slight turning of the head in the direction of the sound. Quieting, listening attitude. 6 months: turns head toward the sound but need not recognize that the sound source is below or above. 8 months: turns head 45° or more in the direction of the sound. Usually determines whether sound source is above or below.*	No response or developmental delay.	Refer all children who demonstrate lack of adequate response for complete audiometric evaluation.

*From Down, M. P., and Silver, H. K.: Clin. Pediatr. **11**:563, Oct. 1972.

Continued.

Physical assessment guide—cont'd

Procedure	Expected findings (age dependent)	Deviations	Implications for health care
		Ears—cont'd	
c. Child and adolescent:			
Determine signs of possible hearing deficit by inadequate performance in school, concern of parents, or speech inadequacy.			All indications of inadequate hearing function require complete audiometric evaluation.
Screen for hearing ability by one of the following methods:			
Rub fingers together quickly in front of each ear for high frequency sound.	Hears fingers rubbing.		
Have child listen to ticking watch.	Hears ticking.		
Weber's test: place tuning fork handle on center of forehead after striking; have child indicate where the sound is heard.	Hears equal sound on each side.		
Rinne test: bone conduction is tested with tuning fork handle placed on mastoid process after striking. Without interfering with sound, the fork is placed near external ear to test air conduction.	Child hears sound in each position; air conduction is longer than bone conduction.	Child is not able to hear with either bone or air conduction tests.	

Physical assessment guide—cont'd

Procedure	Expected findings (age dependent)	Deviations	Implications for health care
	Ears—cont'd		
Child is asked to indicate when the sound disappears in each position.			
	NECK		
1. Palpate trachea, larynx, thyroid, carotid artery, and cervical lymph nodes.	Trachea, larynx, and thyroid are in the midline. Equality of pulsation on each carotid artery. Lymph nodes not palpable.	Enlargements or displacements to one side. Inequality of pulsation. Nodes palpable.	Requires specialist evaluation. Determine adequacy of cardiac and circulatory system. Determine signs of systemic infection.
2. Palpate posterior cervical lymph nodes.	No tenderness. Not palpable.	Tenderness and enlargement of nodes.	Determine other signs of infection or other systemic illness.
3. Appraise position and movement of neck.	Normal position of neck and head. Full range of motion.	Abnormal position. Painful movement.	Administer comfort measures (warmth, massage) for transient muscle strain. Persistent problem requires specialist evaluation.
4. Appraise function of accessory nerve (XI) by having child turn head against opposing pressure on either side and by having child lift shoulders simultaneously against opposing pressure applied by the examiner.	Equality of strength on each side.	Evidence of weakness or atrophy.	Evaluate in light of other neurologic findings.
	CHEST		
1. Measure at the level of the nipples in a plane at right angles to the vertebral crown.	See charts in Chapter 4. Chest may be 1 or 2 cm smaller than head until age 5 months.	Barreling of chest with increased posteroanterior girth.	Determine adequacy of lung function. Requires specialist evaluation.
2. Palpate axillary nodes by closing child's arm against palpating hand, using a rotary motion in the axilla with two or three fingers.	Nodes not palpable.	Presence of enlarged palpable nodes.	Determine other signs of infection or systemic disease.

Continued.

Physical assessment guide—cont'd

Procedure	Expected findings (age dependent)	Deviations	Implications for health care
	CHEST—cont'd		
3. Inspect nipples and breast tissue.	Infancy: some discharge and swelling of breast tissue present in term male and female infants. Puberty: girls begin normal breast development (see p. 84). Boys may exhibit enlargement of breast tissue during adolescence.	Lack of breast tissue indicates prematurity. Delayed development beyond age 16.	Counsel regarding infant's response to maternal hormones. Teaching and counseling regarding physical changes of puberty. Requires specialist evaluation. Reassurance regarding adequacy of sexual development.
	Heart		
1. Percuss chest to estimate heart size and position.	Size and position should be approximately as indicated. 	Enlargement or displacement of heart.	Determine adequacy of cardiac and respiratory systems; specialist evaluation required.
2. Determine the position of the apex beat by palpation of the position closest to the axilla and the lower rib margin.	Infant-2 years: difficult to determine. (Note: the infant heart lies more horizontally with the left border extending to the left of the midclavicle line.) 2-7 years: located in the 4th interspace just to the left of the midclavicle line. Over 7 years: located at the 5th interspace at the midclavicle line.	Positioning indicative of enlargement or displacement.	Requires specialist evaluation.

3. Auscultate heart sounds as follows:
a. Eliminate environmental noise.
b. Ask child to expirate and hold breath when possible.
c. Listen to sounds as indicated:
  1, Aortic.
  2, Pulmonic.
  3, Right ventricular.
  4, Mitral or apical.
	No murmurs.
	Functional murmurs may be present and are generally distinguished as beginning within a very brief interval after the first heart sound and ending well in advance of the second heart sound. The heart sounds themselves are normal. The murmur is usually low-pitched, coarsely "vibratory," and somewhat decrescendo. It is usually heard best at or near the upper left sternal border, 2nd or 3rd interspace.
		Congenital or acquired cardiac pathology, which may be accompanied by any or all of the following:
		Edema.
		Increased respiratory rate.
		Increased heart rate.
		Clubbing of fingers.
		Cold, mottled extremities.
		Periodic anoxia.
		Cyanosis.
			All deviations from normal sounds, including functional murmurs, require specialist evaluation.
			When functional murmur has been defined, family may need counsel regarding meaning and implications of the medical diagnosis.

Physical assessment guide—cont'd

Procedure	Expected findings (age dependent)	Deviations	Implications for health care

Heart—cont'd

5, Xiphoid.

d. Accurately describe timing and characteristics of unusual sounds.

Lungs

Procedure	Expected findings (age dependent)	Deviations	Implications for health care
1. Inspect respiratory movement.	Contoured and symmetrical in both anterior and posterior aspects with slight flaring of the lower costal margin until puberty. Clavicles level, symmetrical. Angle of the lower costal margin is 45° in relation to the sternum.	Splinting. Intercostal, substernal, or other retractions. Prolonged expiratory phase. Excessive flaring of lower margin. "Barreling" of the chest (anteroposterior diameter approaches the lateral diameter). Increased angle.	Inadequacies of respiratory movement indicate full investigation of adequacy of cardiorespiratory system and specialist evaluation.
2. Auscultate breath sound. Compare intensity, pitch, relative duration of inspiratory and expiratory phase, listening from above downward, cross-checking from one side of the chest to the other. Allow two to three breaths in each area. Evaluate sounds during expiration, inhalation, cough, and deep breathing.	Expiratory phase is about twice as long as inspiratory. Only the sound of air moving in and out of lungs should be heard. Sounds are equal in all four quadrants. Four to six uncomplicated upper respiratory tract infections per year are within expected limits for early childhood. See Chapter 6.	Complications of a simple upper respiratory tract infection, including: Rales. Pleural friction "rub." Grunting. Retractions. Wheezing. Post-tussive rales.	Teaching regarding care of child with uncomplicated upper respiratory tract infection (see Chapter 6). Administer skin test for tuberculosis. Complications require specialist evaluation and specific nursing care.

Continued.

Physical assessment guide—cont'd

Procedure	Expected findings (age dependent)	Deviations	Implications for health care
ABDOMEN			
1. Note size, contour, and nature of respiratory movements of abdomen.	Symmetrical contour. Infant-3 years: protuberant abdomen with respiratory movements, particularly during sleep. Over 4 years: Abdomen approximates horizontal plane of chest. No respiratory movements.	Asymmetry of contour. Markedly visible peristalsis. Protuberance with abnormal percussion sounds Visible veins.	Determine adequacy of nutrition and hydration. Determine adequacy of cardiorespiratory system. Deviations require specialist evaluation.
2. Percuss and palpate abdominal organs, particularly liver, spleen, kidneys. Child must be relaxed for effective estimation.	Newborn: liver may be felt 1-2 cm below right costal margin. Tip of spleen may be felt well under left costal margin. Child: liver and spleen are located well under costal margin. No masses or tenderness in any area of the abdomen.	Enlarged organs. Hernia around the umbilicus or in the groin. Appendicitis with localized tenderness as inflammation becomes more severe.	Determine adequacy of all systems. Obtain appropriate blood and urine studies. Obtain specialist evaluation.
3. Auscultate bowel sounds with stethoscope.	Normal bowel sounds are clearly heard every 10-15 seconds with characteristic gentle rumble.	Absence of sounds. Increased sounds.	Determine adequacy of hydration. Treat minor gastrointestinal disturbances per MP (see Chapter 6).
4. Observe umbilicus.	Infant: cord ordinarily dries within 3-5 days and separates by the 14th day. Child: flat to 0.5 cm protrusion; no hernias.	Infection around cord. Patent urachus. Hernia.	Teaching regarding cord care and hygiene. Deviations require specialist evaluation.
5. Palpate femoral pulses just medial to the vertical anterior tendons.	Equal on both sides.	Pulses unequal or absent	Determine adequacy of circulatory system, particularly to lower extremities. Requires specialist evaluation.
BACK AND SPINE			
Observe symmetry and structure of back and spine. Have child stand, walk, sit, and touch toes with fingers from standing position.	Infant: anterior cervical curve begins to develop when the head is held erect at 4-7 weeks. Child: iliac crests equal; scapulae equal; spinal column straight with symmetrical configuration of vertebrae; when bending over, configuration of shoulders symmetrical.	Asymmetry. Incurvation. Scoliosis.	Deviations require specialist evaluation.

Physical assessment guide—cont'd

Procedure	Expected findings (age dependent)	Deviations	Implications for health care
	EXTREMITIES		
1. Inspect arms and legs for:			
a. Edema, color, temperature.	No edema, good color, appropriate skin temperature.	Edema, paleness, coolness.	
b. Lesions, nodules, abnormal pigmentations.	Minor scratches and bruises only.	Major lesions or bruises.	
c. Pulses	Symmetrical, strong pulses.	Absence or asymmetry of pulses.	
d. Features of nailbeds (apply pressure, release, and observe return of coloring).	Blanching with rapid return of color, normal configuration of nails, adequate hygiene.	Clubbing. Delayed return of color after blanching.	Determine adequacy of circulatory system; obtain specialist evaluation.
2. Inspect palmar creases.	Normal configuration.	Transverse line or other unusual crease patterns.	Determine possible signs of congenital malformations; obtain specialist evaluation.
3. Appraise muscle tone, strength, and size by having child squeeze examiner's hands with both hands simultaneously; put extremities through range of active motion against resistance from examiner.	Equal in strength.	Inequality of strength. Loss of strength when the ability was previously observed.	Counseling regarding physical exercise and activity. Deviations require specialist evaluation.
4. Appraise movement and mobility of all joints by observing passive and active range of motion.	Normal range of motion without discomfort.	Limited range of motion. Swelling around joints. Spasticity or catch in muscle associated with sudden relaxation. Rigidity with resistance to muscle movement throughout range of motion.	Deviations require specialist evaluation.
5. Observe ordinary position of comfort of all extremities.	Infant: Extremities flexed while resting. Some bowing of legs may be present because of intrauterine position. As walking and standing begin, normal stance is with toes turned in, knees flexed, and gastrocnemius muscles out.	Extension of extremities. Persistent bowing of legs. Rachitic bowing is usually found at junction of lower and middle thirds of legs, extending anteriorly and laterally.	Deviations require specialist evaluation.

Continued.

Physical assessment guide—cont'd

Procedure	Expected findings (age dependent)	Deviations	Implications for health care
	EXTREMITIES—cont'd		
6. Abduct hips passively while child is on firm surface. Infant: extend index finger along lateral aspect of thigh, palpating hip joint.	Complete 90° abduction without pain or resistance. Equality in gluteal folds.	Limitation of abduction. Pain. Uneven gluteal folds. Ortolani's click in hip joint.	Deviations require specialist evaluation.
7. Observe position of feet.	See p. 16.		
	URINARY SYSTEM		
1. Determine frequency, amount, and characteristics of voiding.	Normal output: 1-6 years—300-600 cc/24 hr. 6-12 years—500-1,500 cc/24 hr. No discomfort with voiding. Stream straight with moderate force. Frequency gradually decreases by age 5 years to 4-6 voidings during waking hours. Toilet training should be accomplished according to cultural and familial preference; usually occurs by 3 years of age with periodic misses during the day until age 4 and night misses until age 5 or 6.	Increased or decreased output. Hematuria. Discomfort with voiding. Stream deflected to one side; weak force. Frequency and urgency. Regression to infantile pattern of toileting after a period of relatively mature habits. Undue anxiety and pressure in family unit regarding toilet training. Persistent night wetting.	Obtain complete urinalysis (see Chapter 4). Determine state of hydration. Determine possible infection. Requires specialist evaluation. Determine adequacy of cardiac and respiratory systems. Deviations require specialist evaluation. Teaching and guidance related to toilet training. Requires specialist evaluation.
2. Obtain urine sample for analysis (see Chapter 4).	No glucose or protein present. Some protein may be found up to 30 minutes after heavy exercise and under orthostatic conditions.	Excessive glucose. Functional disorder of the kidney. Structural disorder. Inflammatory disease.	Determine adequacy of all metabolic systems. Determine family history of diabetes; obtain specialist evaluation. Deviations require specialist evaluation.
3. Note odor of urine.	Nonoffensive, mild odor.	Foul odor. Maple syrup odor. Strong ammonia odor.	Determine signs of infection.

Physical assessment guide—cont'd

Procedure	Expected findings (age dependent)	Deviations	Implications for health care
GENITALIA			
Observe structural adequacy of external genitalia.	GIRLS Symmetrical labia; urinary meatus and vaginal orifice visible. Infant: some bloody discharge may be present during the first 3-4 days in response to maternal hormones. Pubescence: Pubic hair begins to appear. Menses begins (see p. 84).	Anatomic deviations. Irritation from soap, dyes, clothing. Bruises, lacerations, or other signs of abuse. Delayed development. Unusual cramping with menses. Unusual emotional response to changes.	Deviations require specialist evaluation.
	BOYS Normal penis and scrotum with adequate urinary orifice. Circumcision may be present. Testes descended. Pubescence: see p. 84.	Undescended testes. Developmental delay of secondary sexual characteristics. Irritation of genitalia from infection or abuse.	Deviations require specialist evaluation.
ANUS			
Determine patency and normal configuration.	Symmetrical.	Fissures. Stenosis. Hemorrhoids. Pinworms.	Teaching regarding adequate hygiene and bowel habits. Deviations may require specialist evaluation.

CHAPTER 3

Assessment of learning and thought, social, and inner competencies

A complete nursing assessment includes data from the physical examination, history, interview, and direct observation of behavior; these data provide information related to the child's learning and thought, social, and inner competencies. This chapter presents general descriptions of assessment data that are used for various stages of development and provides guidelines for interpretation of these data. However, definitive descriptions of competencies in these areas of development are not available, and interpretation of each child's development must be made within the context of the child's family and cultural expectations and with an understanding of the wide range of normal behaviors that can occur within each cultural group.

Learning and thought competency is the child's ability to use complex mental powers to perform those operations that are deemed to be unique human cognitive traits. Understanding and using language, reasoning, solving increasingly complex problems, giving cognitive attention to affective dimensions of human existence, idealizing, fantasizing, and giving mental projection into the future are among the many learning and thought traits acquired during the years of growth and development. Table 4-9 (pp. 67-72) presents normative values for assessment of receptive and expressive language abilities. The Peabody Picture Vocabulary Test* is a useful screening tool for estimating verbal intelligence ability of middle-class English-speaking children. Children's drawings of persons can provide a rough estimate of intellectual maturity†; however, standardized tests of intelligence and tests of academic aptitude and achievement are usually preferred. Factors in the environment that influence learning and thought competency are considered for each stage of development. The outlined material below presents guidelines for assessment of caretaker behaviors that influence learning and thought competency during infancy and during the toddler period. During the preschool, school-age, and adolescent periods the school environment is assessed for adequacy in promoting the child's learning and thought competency.

_____
*Dunn, L. M.: Peabody Picture Vocabulary Test, Minneapolis, 1965, American Guidance Service, Inc.
†Harns, D. B.: Children's drawings as measures of intellectual maturity, New York, 1963, Harcourt Brace Jovanovich, Inc.

**ASSESSMENT OF CARE-GIVER BEHAVIORS
THAT STIMULATE LEARNING AND THOUGHT
COMPETENCY DURING INFANCY***

I. Language facilitation
  A. Elicits vocalization (through initiation and contingent responses)
  B. Converses; chats to infant
  C. Praises or encourages infant
  D. Offers help or solicitous remarks
  E. Inquires of child; requests
  F. Gives explanation, information, cultural rules
  G. Labels sensory experiences
  H. Reads or shows pictures to child
  I. Sings to or plays music for child
II. Social-emotional positive inputs
  A. Smiles at infant
  B. Uses loving or reassuring tones
  C. Provides loving physical contact
  D. Plays social games with infant
  E. Uses eye contact to arouse, orient, or sustain infant's attention
III. Social-emotional negative inputs
  A. Criticizes verbally; scolds
  B. Forbids; gives negative commands
  C. Acts angry; is physically impatient; frowns; restrains infant
  D. Punishes physically
  E. Isolates child for unacceptable behaviors
  F. Ignores child when child shows need for attention
IV. Presentation of planned learning games
  A. Presents "things don't disappear" games
  B. Presents "using a tool" games
  C. Presents activities that use imitation
  D. Presents "cause it to happen" games
  E. Makes use of space (as in nesting and stacking games and detour games)
  F. Presents handling and pickup games
  G. Introduces new games appropriate to developmental changes
V. Care-giving routines with child
  A. Feeds
  B. Diapers; toilets
  C. Dresses; undresses
  D. Washes; cleans
  E. Prepares infant for sleep
  F. Provides physical shepherding
  G. Eye-checks on infant's well-being
VI. Care-giving routines with environment
  A. Prepares food
  B. Tidies room or environment
  C. Helps other caregivers
VII. Physical development
  A. Provides kinesthetic stimulation
  B. Provides large-muscle play

Assessment of social and inner competencies is closely related during each stage of development. Social competency includes a description of the nature and quality of the child's interactions with significant others as well as with strangers, and these experiences provide the foundation for the child's development of inner competency or the inner perceptions that the child develops regarding the self. The Vineland Social Maturity Scale* may be used to obtain an objective estimate of social maturity during early childhood and the school-age periods. Table 3-1 presents a summary of behavior characteristics and psychopathology in parent-child relationships. Table 3-2 presents a summary of behavior problems during early childhood and guidelines for differentiating between expected or normal behavior and problem behavior during this developmental stage. Infants and young children who experience a threatened or real loss (for example, parental separation or divorce, death) are at a particular risk for poor social and inner competency development. Table 3-3 presents guidelines for estimating the extent of risk for such a child and the intervention that is recommended for these children. Tables 3-4 and 3-5 present interview guidelines for assessment of the inner competency of school-age children and adolescents.

Detailed description of the assessment of these competencies is found in *Child Health Maintenance: Concepts in Family-Centered Care*, Chapters 9, 10, 11, and 13.

---

*Adapted from Honig, A. S., and Lally, J. R.: Assessing teacher behaviors with infants in day care. In Friedlander, B. Z., Sterritt, G. M., and Kirk, G. E., editors: Exceptional infant, vol. 3, New York, 1975, Brunner/Mazel, Inc., p. 533.

---

*Doll, E. A.: Vineland Social Maturity Scale, Circle Pines, Minn., 1965, American Guidance Service, Inc.

Table 3-1. Behavior characteristics and psychopathology in parent-child relationships*

Tasks in process	Acceptable behavior characteristics	Minimal psychopathology	Extreme psychopathology
NEWBORN AND YOUNG INFANT (BIRTH TO 6 MONTHS)			
Infant			
To adjust physiologically to extrauterine life To develop appropriate psychologic response To assimilate experientially, with increasing capacity to postpone and accept substitutes	Copes with mechanics of life (eating, sleeping, etc.) Body needs urgent Reflexes dominate Establishes symbiotic relationship to mother Sucking behavior predominant Cries when distressed Responds to mouth, skin, sense modalities Functions egocentrically Is completely dependent Low patience tolerance Needs expressed instinctively Develops trust in adult	Feeding and digestive problems Sleep disturbances Excessive sucking activity Excessive motor discharge Excessive crying Excessive irritability Difficult to comfort	Lethargy (depression) Marasmus Cannot be comforted Unresponsive Infantile autism Developmental arrest
Mother			
To sustain baby and self physically and pleasurably To give and get emotional gratification from nurturing To foster and integrate baby's development	Provides feeding and fondling Gets to know baby Has tolerance for baby Promotes sense of trust Learns baby's cues Interacts emotionally with baby Encourages baby's development Has reasonable expectations of baby Develops good working relationship with baby	Indifference to baby Ambivalence toward baby and its needs Self-doubt and anxiety Intolerance of baby's characteristics Overresponds or underresponds to baby Premature or inappropriate expectations Dissatisfaction with role of motherhood	Alienation from baby Severe depression Excessive guilt Complete inability to function in maternal role Overwhelming and incapacitating anxiety Denies or tries to control baby's needs Severe clashes with baby Vents dissatisfactions on baby
OLDER INFANT (6 TO 18 MONTHS)			
Infant			
To develop more reliance and self-control To differentiate self from mother To make developmental progress	More stable physiologically Increased voluntary motor activity and exploration Higher level of patience tolerance Instinctual needs in better control Strong selective tie to mother Stranger differentiation Increased play, verbalizing, and sensorimotor behavior Discernible social responses	Excessive crying, anger, and irritability Low frustration tolerance Excessive negativism Finicky eater, sleep disturbances Digestive and elimination problems Distinctive motility patterns (rocking, etc.) Delayed development	Frequent tantrums Apathy, immobility, withdrawal Extreme, obsessive fingersucking, rocking, headbanging No interest in objects, play, or environment Anorexia Psychogenic megacolon Inexpressive of feelings No social discrimination No tie to mother; wary of all adults Infantile autism

*From Rudolf, A. M., editor: Pediatrics, ed. 16, New York, 1977, Appleton-Century-Crofts; pp. 20-23.

Table 3-1. Behavior characteristics and psychopathology in parent-child relationships—cont'd

Tasks in process	Acceptable behavior characteristics	Minimal psychopathology	Extreme psychopathology
OLDER INFANT (6 TO 18 MONTHS)—cont'd			
Infant—cont'd			
	Outbursts of negativism and anger		Failure to thrive
	Sensory modalities important		Arrested development
	Emergence of idiosyncratic patterns		
	Demonstrates memory and anticipation		
	Begins to imitate		
Mother			
To provide a healthy physical and emotional climate	Satisfaction from serving baby	Disappointed in and unaccepting of baby	Neglect or abuse of baby
To foster weaning, training, habits	Responds appropriately to baby's signs of distress	Misses baby's cues	Rejection of the maternal role
To understand, appreciate, and accept baby	Aware of baby's inborn reaction pattern	Infancy unappealing	Severe hostility reactions
	Has more confidence in own ability	Impersonal management	No attempt to understand or gratify baby
	Gives positive psychologic reassurances (fondling, talking)	Attempts to coerce to desired behavior	Deliberately thwarts baby
	Shows pleasure in baby	Overanxious or overprotective	Complete withdrawal and separation from baby
	Keeps pace with baby's advances	Mildly depressed or apathetic	
	Accepts baby's idiosyncrasies		
TODDLER AND PRESCHOOL AGE (UNDER 5 YEARS)			
Child			
To reach physiologic plateaus (motor action, toilet training)	Gratification from exercise of neuromotor skills	Poor motor coordination	Extreme lethargy, passivity, or hypermotility
To differentiate self and secure sense of autonomy	Investigative, imitative, imaginative play	Persistent speech problems	Little or no speech; noncommunicative
To tolerate separations from mother	Actions somewhat modified by thought	Timidity toward people and experiences	No response or relationship to people; symbiotic clinging to mother
To develop conceptual frames and ethical values	Memory good; original thinking	Fears and night terrors	Somatic ills; vomiting, constipation, diarrhea, tics
To master instinctual psychologic impulses (oedipal, sexual, guilt)	Exercises autonomy with body (sphincter control; eating)	Problems with eating, sleeping, elimination, toileting, weaning	Autism; childhood psychosis
To assimilate and handle socialization and acculturation (aggression relationships, feelings)	Dependence on mother and separation fears	Irritability, crying, temper tantrums	Excessive enuresis, fecal soiling, fears
To learn sex distinctions	Behavior identification with parents, siblings, peers	Partial return to infantile manners	Completely infantile behavior
	Learns speech for communication	Inability to leave mother without panic	Play inhibited or nonconceptualized; absence or excess of autoerotic behavior
	Awareness of own motives, beginnings of conscience	Fear of strangers	Obsessive-compulsive behavior, ritual mannerisms
	Intense feelings of shame, guilt, joy, desire to please	Breath-holding spells	Impulsive destructive behavior
	Standards of good and bad	Lack of interest in other children	
	Sex curiosity and differentiation		

Continued.

Table 3-1. Behavior characteristics and psychopathology in parent-child relationships—cont'd

Tasks in process	Acceptable behavior characteristics	Minimal psychopathology	Extreme psychopathology
TODDLER AND PRESCHOOL AGE (UNDER 5 YEARS)—cont'd			
Child—cont'd			
	Dependence, independence, ambivalence		
	Questions birth and death		
Mother			
To promote training, habits	Moderate and flexible in training	Premature, coercive, or censoring training	Severely coercive, punitive
To aid family and group socialization of child	Shows pleasure and praise for child's advances	Exacting standards above child's ability to conform	Totally critical and rejecting
To encourage speech and other learning	Encourages and participates with child's ability to play	Transmits anxiety and tension	Overidentification with or overly submissive to child
To reinforce child's sense of autonomy and identity	Sets reasonable standards and controls	Unaccepting of child's efforts, intolerant toward failure	Severe repression of child's need for gratification
To set a model for ethical conduct	Paces herself to child's capacity	Overreacts, overprotective, overanxious	Deprivation of all stimulations, freedoms, and pleasures
To delineate male and female roles	Consistent in own behavior, conduct, and ethics	Despondent, apathetic	Extreme anger and displeasure with child
	Provides emotional reassurance to child		Child assault and abuse
	Promotes peer play and guided group activity		Severe depression and withdrawal
	Reinforces child's cognition of male and female roles		
SCHOOL AGE AND PREADOLESCENCE (5 TO 12 YEARS)			
Child			
To master greater physical prowess	General good health, greater body competence, acute sensory perception	Anxiety and oversensitivity to new experiences (school, relationships, separation)	Extreme withdrawal, apathy, depression, grief, self-destructive tendencies
To further establish self-identity and sex role	Pride and self-confidence; less dependence on parents	Lack of attentiveness, learning difficulties, disinterest in learning	Complete failure to learn
To work toward greater independence from parents	Better impulse control	Acting-out: lying, stealing, temper outbursts; inappropriate social behavior	Speech difficulty, especially stuttering
To become aware of world at large	Ambivalence re dependency, separation, and new experiences	Regressive behavior (wetting, soiling, crying, fears)	Extreme and uncontrollable antisocial behavior (aggression, destruction, chronic lying, stealing, intentional cruelty to animals)
To develop peer and other relationships	Accepts own sex role; psychosexual expression in play and fantasy	Appearance of compulsive mannerisms (tics, rituals)	
To acquire learning, new skills, and a sense of industry	Equates parents with peers and other adults	Somatic illness: eating and sleeping problems, aches, pains, digestive upsets	Severe obsessive-compulsive behavior (phobias, fantasies, rituals)
	Aware of natural world (life, death, birth, science); subjective but realistic world	Fear of illness and body injury	Inability to distinguish reality from fantasy
	Competitive but well organized in play; enjoys peer interaction	Difficulties and rivalry with peers, siblings, adults; constant fighting	Excessive sexual exhibitionism, eroticism, sexual assaults on others
	Regard for collective obedience to social laws, rules, and fair play	Destructive tendencies strong; temper tantrums	Extreme somatic illness: failure to thrive, anorexia, obesity, hypochondriasis, abnormal menses

Table 3-1. Behavior characteristics and psychopathology in parent-child relationships—cont'd

Tasks in process	Acceptable behavior characteristics	Minimal psychopathology	Extreme psychopathology
SCHOOL AGE AND PREADOLESCENCE (5 TO 12 YEARS)—cont'd			
Child—cont'd			
	Explores environment; school and neighborhood basic to social learning experience Cognition advancing; intuitive thinking advancing to concrete operational level; responds to teaching Speech becomes reasoning and expressive tool; thinking still egocentric	Inability or unwillingness to do things for self Moodiness and withdrawal; few friends or personal relationships	Complete absence or deterioration of personal and peer relationships
Parents			
To help child's emancipation from parents To reinforce self-identification and independence To provide positive pattern of social and sex role behavior To acclimatize child to world at large To facilitate learning, reasoning, communication, and experiencing To promote wholesome moral and ethical values	Ambivalent toward child's separation but encourage independence Mixed feelings about parent-surrogates, but help child to accept them Encourage child to participate outside of home Set appropriate model of social and ethical behavior and standards Take pleasure in child's developing skills and abilities Understand and cope with child's behavior Find other gratifications in life (activity, employment) Supportive toward child as required	Disinclination to separate from child; or prematurely hastening separation Signs of despondency, apathy, hostility Foster fears, dependence, apprehension Disinterested in or rejecting of child Overly critical and censuring; undermine child's confidence Inconsistent in discipline or control; erratic in behavior Offer a restrictive, overly moralistic model	Extreme depression and withdrawal; rejection of child Intense hostility; aggression toward child Uncontrollable fears, anxieties, guilts Complete inability to function in family role Severe moralistic prohibition of child's independent strivings

Continued.

Table 3-1. Behavior characteristics and psychopathology in parent-child relationships—cont'd

Tasks in process	Acceptable behavior characteristics	Minimal psychopathology	Extreme psychopathology
PUBERTY AND EARLY ADOLESCENCE (12 TO 15 YEARS) **Child**			
To come to terms with body changes	Heightened physical power, strength, and coordination	Apprehensions, fears, guilt, and anxiety re sex, health, education	Complete withdrawal into self, extreme depression
To cope with sexual development and psychosexual drives	Occasional psychosomatic and somatopsychic disturbances	Defiant, negative, impulsive, or depressed behavior	Acts of delinquency, asceticism, ritualism, overconformity
To establish and confirm sense of identity	Maturing sex characteristics and proclivities	Frequent somatic or hypochondriacal complaints, or denial of ordinary illnesses	Neuroses, especially phobias; persistent anxiety, compulsions, inhibitions, or constrictive behavior
To learn further re sex role	Review and resolution of oedipal conflicts		Persistent hypochondriases
To synthesize personality	Inconsistent, unpredictable, and paradoxical behavior	Learning irregular or deficient	Sex aberrations
To struggle for independence and emancipation from family	Exploration and experimentation with self and world	Sexual preoccupation	Somatic illness: anorexia, colitis, menstrual disorders
To incorporate learning to the gestalt of living	Eagerness for peer approval and relationships	Poor or absent personal relationships with adults or peers	Complete inability to socialize or work (learning, etc.)
	Strong moral and ethical perceptions	Immaturity or precocious behavior; unchanging personality and temperament	Psychoses
	Cognitive development accelerated; deductive and inductive reasoning; operational thought	Unwillingness to assume responsibility of greater autonomy	
	Competitive in play; erratic work-play patterns	Inability to substitute or postpone gratifications	
	Better use of language and other symbolic material		
	Critical of self and others; self-evaluative		
	Highly ambivalent toward parents		
	Anxiety over loss of parental nurturing		
	Hostility to parents		
	Verbal aggression		

Table 3-1. Behavior characteristics and psychopathology in parent-child relationships—cont'd

Tasks in process	Acceptable behavior characteristics	Minimal psychopathology	Extreme psychopathology
PUBERTY AND EARLY ADOLESCENCE (12 TO 15 YEARS)—cont'd			
Parents			
To help child complete emancipation	Allow and encourage reasonable independence	Sense of failure	Severe depression and withdrawal
To provide support and understanding	Set fair rules; be consistent	Disappointment greater than joy	Complete rejection of child and/or family
To limit child's behavior and set standards	Compassionate and understanding; firm but not punitive or derogatory	Indifference to child and family	Inability to function in family role
To offer favorable and appropriate environment for healthy development	Feel pleasure and pride, occasional guilt and disappointment	Apathy and depression	Rivalrous, competitive, destructive, and abusive to child
To recall own adolescent difficulties; to accept and respect the adolescent's differences or similarities to parents or others	Have other interests besides child	Persistent intolerence of child	Abetting child's acting-out of unacceptable sexual or aggressive impulses for vicarious reasons
To relate to adolescents and adolescence with a constructive sense of humor	Marital life fulfilled apart from child	Limited interests and self-expression	Perpetuation of incapacitating infantilism in the preadolescent
	Occasional expression of intolerance, resentment, envy, or anxiety about adolescent's development	Loss of perspective about child's capacities	Panic reactions to acceptable standards of sexual behavior, social activity, and assertiveness
		Occasional direct or vicarious reversion to adolescent impulses	Compulsive, obsessive, or psychotic behavior
		Uncertainty about standards regarding sexual behavior and deviant social or personal activity	

Table 3-2. Summary of behavior problems during early childhood, normal expectations, and factors that contribute to problem behavior

Behavior	Normal expectations	Factors that contribute to problem behavior	
		Child factors	Parent/home environment factors
Sleep disorders	Occasional nightmares beginning at about 36 months. Ritual bedtime routine; attempt to delay sleep peaks between 2-3 years. Head banging and rocking between 1-4 years providing release of tension. Waking between 1 and 5 AM occurs infrequently after 6 months of age (less than once a week). Fearful of darkness between 2-5 years; will settle down with use of rituals, such as having a favorite toy or a night-light.	Excessive napping during the day. Insufficient adult interaction during the day, leading to use of bedtime as opportunity to gain adult attention. Unusual fears related to darkness, being left alone; rituals and night-light do not suffice. Illness. Development of nighttime bowel and bladder control.	Anxiety for child's safety results in frequent checking on child, disturbing sleep. Inability to set and maintain limits on delaying tactics. Unrealistic expectations; cannot tolerate bedtime rituals. Environment noisy, not conducive to sleep. Excessive stimulation before bedtime. Frightening TV shows before bedtime. Environmental stress such as new sibling, move, and so on.
Temper tantrums	Tantrums peak at 2 years of age, decreasing in frequency and intensity until they rarely occur by about 4 years of age. Usually occur in response to frustrated desires of a child, such as wanting a toy that cannot be purchased.	Used as a manipulative device to gain control of parental behavior. Insufficient positive interaction with adults, leading to use of tantrums to gain attention.	Inability to set and maintain limits; parents allow themselves to be manipulated. Insufficient positive approaches to child in response to desired behavior. Unrealistic expectations; cannot tolerate any tantrum behavior.
Toilet training and bed-wetting	Child has full physiologic capacity for day control by 3 years, night control by 4 years. Daytime and nighttime "accidents" occur throughout early childhood, decreasing in frequency by 4-5 years. Regression occurs with environmental or social changes, such as arrival of sibling, moving, divorce.	Fears and anxiety in response to negative means of toilet training inhibit ability to gain control. Used as an attention-getting device if positive means of gaining attention are lacking. Excessive fluid intake before bedtime.	Punishment and other negative approaches to toilet training. Unrealistic expectations for control; expect normal control before physiologic ability is present, or expect the child to be accident-free. Inconsistent recognition of child's signals of needing to use the toilet. Inadequate provision for child's toileting needs, such as small commode. Clothing is too difficult for child to maneuver independently. Irregular eating patterns.

Table 3-2. Summary of behavior problems during early childhood, normal expectations, and factors that contribute to problem behavior—cont'd

Behavior	Normal expectations	Factors that contribute to problem behavior	
		Child factors	Parent/home environment factors
Aggressive or quarrelsome behavior; sibling rivalry	Ability to play cooperatively begins to emerge at 4-5 years. Before this age, child is seldom able to share toys; often wants toys that another child has. Predominant use of physical hitting, shoving to express displeasure; verbal abilities begin to emerge during fifth year.	Insufficient positive adult attention leads to deliberate use of aggression to gain adult attention. Aggression may arise from actual or perceived adult preference for sibling or playmate.	Insufficient positive interaction in response to desired behavior. Unrealistic expectations for cooperative and sharing behavior. Actual preferential attention given to sibling or playmate.
Inability to separate; excessive shyness	Child can separate easily by 3 years if the surroundings are consistent, predictable, positive. Continues to protest separation if the environment changes or if confronted by total strangers. Shy in new and strange surroundings; relaxed and spontaneous in familiar surroundings.	Inadequate establishment of self-concept, leading to lack of confidence even in familiar surroundings. Uses protest of separation as a manipulative control device. Fear of being abandoned.	Parental anxiety and guilt over separation. Inability to set limits, to leave child after brief, direct explanation. Lack of preparation for an anticipated separation, leading to an unpredicted, fearful experience for the child. Inconsistent messages and actions, such as telling the child the parent will stay and then sneaking out, or not returning at a predicted time.

Table 3-3. Assessment and intervention for infants and young children who experience stress of threatened or real loss

Assessment factor	Minimal risk	Maximum risk	Resources for minimizing risk
Quality of early mother-child attachment	Solid attachment bond formed.	Early attachment failure or inadequacy; neglect or abuse.	Provide support for existing attachment relationship throughout period of reintegration. _or_ Provide a new attachment figure, maintaining long-term consistency in the relationship.
Family relationships	Family relationships predominantly harmonious before stress event.	Long-term history of family discord, frequent absence of significant member(s).	Provide support for the reestablishment of satisfying family life after stress event. _or_ Provide alternate family environment with predominantly harmonious relationships.
Mental health of parents	Parents mature, well adjusted, have positive outlook, predominantly happy with life before stress event.	Previous incidence of parental depression, withdrawal, or other psychiatric illness.	Provide intervention for mental health problem. Provide a therapeutic relationship for the child with an adult who has adequate mental health.
Information child receives about the stress event	Child is given direct, honest information appropriate to age and in accord with family's religious beliefs and values.	Information withheld from child. Inaccurate information conveyed. Information is distorted to place blame on child.	Counsel family regarding the information needs of the child. Institute direct therapeutic counseling with young child to uncover child's perceptions of the information received, and support the development of reality-based perceptions.
Reactions of other family members to stress event	Periods of initial shock, personal disintegration, and reintegration proceed to unfold within the following year.	Inadequate initial coping, prolonged period of personal disintegration, failure of signs of reintegration.	Long-term therapy for members in personal difficulty. Short-term therapeutic support for minimal risk family members. Therapeutic, secure relationship for child with an adult not involved personally in the stressful experience.

Table 3-4. Interview for nursing assessment of later childhood inner competency

Area of function	Interview questions	Optimal responses
Self-evaluation	1. What do you like best/worst about yourself? 2. If you could change something about yourself, what would it be? 3. How are you like your mother/father? 4. Who is your best friend? What do you like best about him/her? Why does he/she like you?	During the early school-age period the child will be more closely identified with parents, but identification will begin to shift to peers as the school-age period progresses. Identification with peers and parents of the same sex is typical and reflects culturally acquired perceptions of appropriate sex-role behavior. The child's responses should be predominantly positive; some flexibility will be observed, depending on varying situations, but the child will tend to focus on one or two major themes in describing the self. The child's responses should be consistent with the observed behavior of the child.
Prediction of success or failure	1. What would you like to be when you grow up? Why? 2. What is your best/worst subject in school?	School-age children will identify an idealized adult role for themselves that is often based on the role of an admired adult, such as parents, teachers, or TV and movie stars. They will not yet be able to use an assessment of their own abilities in predicting future roles but can associate activities they prefer with the idealized adult role. Their identification of best and worst subjects in school should be accurate and reflect an area of performance that gives personal satisfaction and feelings of success and mastery.
Obtaining personal survival, acceptance, comfort, enhancement, competence, and actualization	1. What do you worry about? What do you do to make yourself feel better? 2. When you have a problem in school, how do you work it out? 3. How do you spend your spare time?	School-age children can identify personal worries and usually have some means of diversion to alleviate preoccupation with worry. They can describe activities and relationships with parents, teachers, or peers that they use to work out problems in school. Spare time should be spent in hobbies and physical activities that reflect a predominance in developing relationships with peers as well as in developing individual interests and abilities.
Instigation of behavior mediated by either one's own desires and values or by society's desires and values	1. How can you tell what is right and wrong? 2. If your friend did something that you think is wrong, what would you do?	During the early school-age period right and wrong are defined by rigid rules that the child has learned from parents, church, or school. As later childhood progresses, situational variables begin to enter into the interpretation of right and wrong, and multiple factors can be taken into account. The young school-age child will be more concerned with justice and punishment for wrongdoing according to culturally defined rules for behavior; later a sense of rehabilitating the wrongdoer and a sense of personal responsibility for behavior emerge.

Table 3-5. Interview for nursing assessment of adolescent inner competency

Area of function	Interview questions	Optimal responses
Self-evaluation	1. How would you describe yourself? 2. What do you like best/worst about yourself? 3. If you could change something about your body right now, what would it be? 4. How are you like your mother/father? 5. What do your friends think of you?	Teenagers can take into account many factors in responding; they should be able to explore and reflect on various dimensions and how they interact. The responses should be consistent with the observed behavior, relatively positive and favorable, and flexible in describing different dimensions of the self suited to different situations.
Prediction of success or failure	1. Tell me about your plans after high school. 2. What can you do best? How do you think you might use this in the future? 3. What is the most difficult thing that you have to do?	Plans for the future should begin to take shape at about 15-16 years; teenagers' expectations should be realistic, taking into account each factor affecting their plans, such as finances, family preferences, peer influences, and ability of the self. Responses should focus on goals and means that assure realistic success.
Obtaining personal survival, acceptance, comfort, enhancement, competence, and actualization	1. What is the biggest problem you have ever had with a friend? How did you work it out? 2. In what ways do you agree/disagree with your parents? 3. How do you spend your spare time? 4. What do you like best/least about school?	Teenagers can identify an interpersonal problem and resolution of the problem. The resolution should indicate taking the other person's point of view into account and some degree of compromise. There are areas of agreement and disagreement with parents and at school; these should not pose a threat to the teenager. Spare time is valued for pleasant, desired, and positive activity.
Instigation of behavior mediated by either one's own desires and values or by society's desires and values	1. Who influences you the most, and why? 2. Have you ever made a decision completely on your own? What was it? What happened? 3. What would you do differently if you were completely on your own? Why?	The primary influence should come from peers or adults outside of the family, although dimensions of family influence should be acknowledged and viewed as relatively positive. Decisions should be motivated from inner desires predominantly. There is a sense of wanting complete independence, but the transient state of dependence on the family is viewed as necessary and not unduly constricting.

CHAPTER 4

Norms and standards for nursing assessment and intervention

The purpose of this chapter is to provide norms and standards useful in the nursing assessment and in planning intervention. Where indicated, instructions for standardized methods for obtaining the data are given, or information regarding where standardized instructions can be obtained is provided. Included in this chapter are:

Instructions for measurement of body size and physical growth, pp. 51-53

Growth charts for girls birth to 18 years, Figs. 4-3 and 4-4, p. 54

Growth charts for boys birth to 18 years, Figs. 4-5 and 4-6, p. 55

Head circumference for girls birth to 36 months, Fig. 4-7, p. 56

Head circumference for boys birth to 36 months, Fig. 4-8, p. 57

Physical growth of black girls, Fig. 4-9, p. 58

Physical growth of black boys, Fig. 4-10, p. 59

Nomogram for estimation of body surface area, Fig. 4-11, p. 59

Classification of newborns by birth weight and gestational age, Fig. 4-12, p. 60

Chest circumference tables, Tables 4-1 to 4-3, pp. 61-62

Pulse rate table, Table 4-4, p. 63

Respiratory rate table, Table 4-5, p. 63

Body temperature table, Table 4-6, p. 64

Blood pressure table, Table 4-7, p. 64

Normal values for laboratory testing of blood and urine, pp. 64-66

Denver Developmental Screening Test, Fig. 4-13, pp. 67-68

Language development table, Table 4-9, pp. 69-72

Denver Articulation Screening Exam, Fig. 4-14, pp. 73-74

Landmarks of visual development, Table 4-10, p. 75

Denver Eye Screening Test, Table 4-11, p. 76

Procedure for Snellen vision screening, pp. 77-78

Preschool Readiness Experimental Screening Scale (PRESS), pp. 79-81

Immunization schedules, Tables 4-12 and 4-13, p. 82

Schedule for preventive dental health care, Table 4-14, pp. 82-84

Developmental states of secondary sex characteristics, Table 4-15, p. 84

Environmental standards, Table 4-16, p. 85

INSTRUCTIONS FOR MEASUREMENT OF BODY SIZE AND PHYSICAL GROWTH*

Measurement of physical growth is a key element in evaluating the health of children. Measurements of length or stature and weight pro-

*Prepared by and adapted from the Preventable Diseases and Nutrition Activity, Bureau of Smallpox Eradication, Center for Disease Control, and The Maternal and Child Health Program, Bureau of Community Health Services, Health Services Administration, Public Health Service, Department of Health, Education, and Welfare.

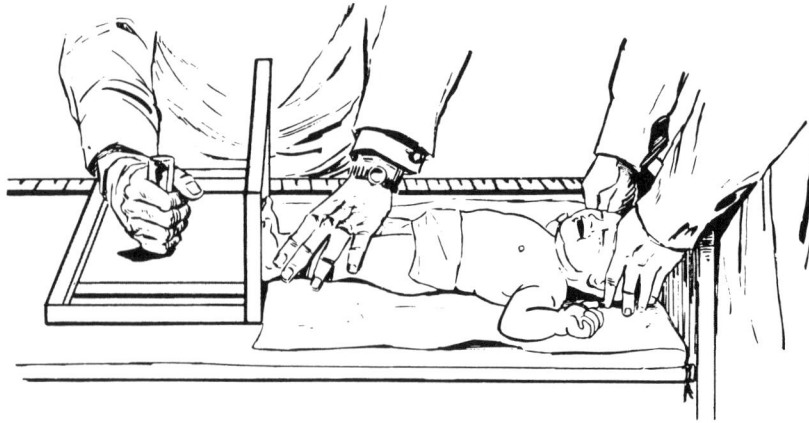

Fig. 4-1. Length measurement of the infant. (From U.S. Department of Health, Education, and Welfare, Public Health Service, Center for Disease Control, Atlanta, Ga.)

vide by far the most useful information. To be of greatest usefulness, these measurements must be accurately made and recorded and compared with appropriate reference data.

How to measure

Length

Until a child is 24 months old he or she should be measured lying on his or her back. From 24 to 36 months, the child may be measured either recumbent or standing, with care taken that the appropriate growth chart be used for recording the results: the chart for 0 to 36 months if supine and for 2 to 18 years if standing. Satisfactory measurement of recumbent length requires adequate equipment (Fig. 4-1) and two examiners. One person holds the child's head in alignment with the body, with the line of vision straight up, and applies gentle traction to bring the top of the head into contact with the fixed headboard. The other person holds the child's feet with toes straight up, pushes down on the knees, and brings the movable footboard to rest firmly against the heels (Fig. 4-1). An examining table can be inexpensively modified to provide a suitable measuring apparatus. Alternatively, a portable measuring board can be constructed.

In measuring length at birth and in early infancy, extension of the legs presents a special problem. The recommended technique is as follows: after placing the infant on the back, bring the knees together, and, pushing down on them, extend the legs fully. Lifting the body slightly with the help of the assistant (to ease the strain on tissues produced by compression at the knees), orient the infant so that the head, with gaze upward, remains in alignment with the body and the crown of the head makes firm contact with the fixed headboard. The assistant holds the head in position while the measurer uses one hand to keep the infant from spreading or flexing the knees and the other hand to bring the movable footboard against the heels.

Stature

All children over 36 months old should be measured standing (Fig. 4-2). A child from 24 to 36 months may be measured either recumbent or standing, with care taken that the appropriate chart be used for recording the results.

The child measured standing should be told to stand up straight and tall and look straight ahead so that the line of vision is perpendicular to the axis of the fully extended body. . . . Do *not* try to measure stature with the movable measuring rod of platform scales. Instead, fix a measuring stick or tape to a true vertical flat surface, either a wall or a rigid, free-standing measuring device. The child should stand on a horizontal bare floor or platform with bare heels close together, almost touching, with back as straight as possible, with heels, buttocks, and back of shoulders touching the wall or vertical surface of the measuring device, and with the line of vision straight ahead. A block, squared at right angles against the wall, should then be brought to the crown of the head and the measurement noted (Fig. 4-2). When an assistant is available, this person should place one hand against the child's knees to detect any flexion of the lower limbs and the other hand on the upper surfaces of the child's feet to detect any lifting of the heels from firm contact with the floor or platform. Length or stature should be measured to the nearest eighth inch, or 1 millimeter.

Weight

Using an appropriate-sized beam balance or scale with nondetachable weights, measure body weight to the nearest half ounce, or 10 grams, for infants, or to the nearest quarter pound, or 100 grams, for children. At least two or three times a year check the accuracy of scales with calibrated or standard weights.* Measurements of weight should be made at a comfortable environmental temperature; infants should be nude and older children clothed only in underpants or a light cotton gown. Every effort should be made to protect children from embarrassment. The child's record should specify special conditions of weighing; the approximate weight of any additional clothing should be indicated or a statement made that weight of such clothing was deducted before the body weight was recorded.

Head circumference

Head circumference, an important screening measurement for micro- or macrocephaly due to nonnutritional abnormalities, may be measured in children up to 36 months old. Since the growth of head circumference up to 2 years of age is so closely related to body length, head circumference measurements add no more information about child nutritional status than do body length measurements. Therefore, head circumference is not a useful screening measure

---

*A dealer in scales will generally be willing to calibrate the balance at intervals. Standard 5- and 10-kg weights can be obtained from the Toledo Scales Co., Toledo, Ohio, or from the Douglas HOMS Co., Inc., Burlingame, Calif.

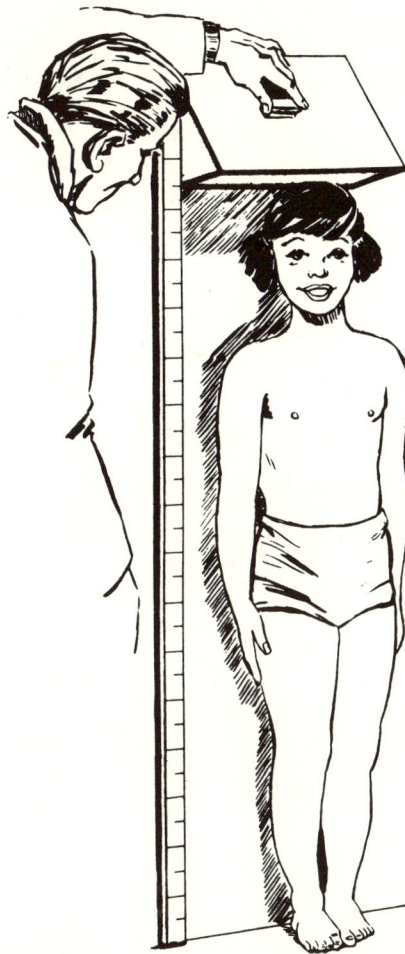

Fig. 4-2. Stature measurement of the child. (From U.S. Department of Health, Education, and Welfare, Public Health Service, Center for Disease Control, Atlanta, Ga.)

for undernutrition when body length is known. Use a nonstretchable, flexible tape, preferably with a slot through which the end passes and a "window" for taking readings. This kind of tape conforms readily to the contours of a child's head and is more easily read.

Apply the tape snugly around the biggest part of the head. It should pass just above the ridges over the eyebrows, just above the insertion of the outer ears, and around the occipital prominence at the back of the head to measure the maximum circumference. It should be pulled tight enough to crush the hair as much as possible. Readings are to the nearest eighth inch, or 1 millimeter.

Growth Charts for U.S. Girls

Name

Birth date

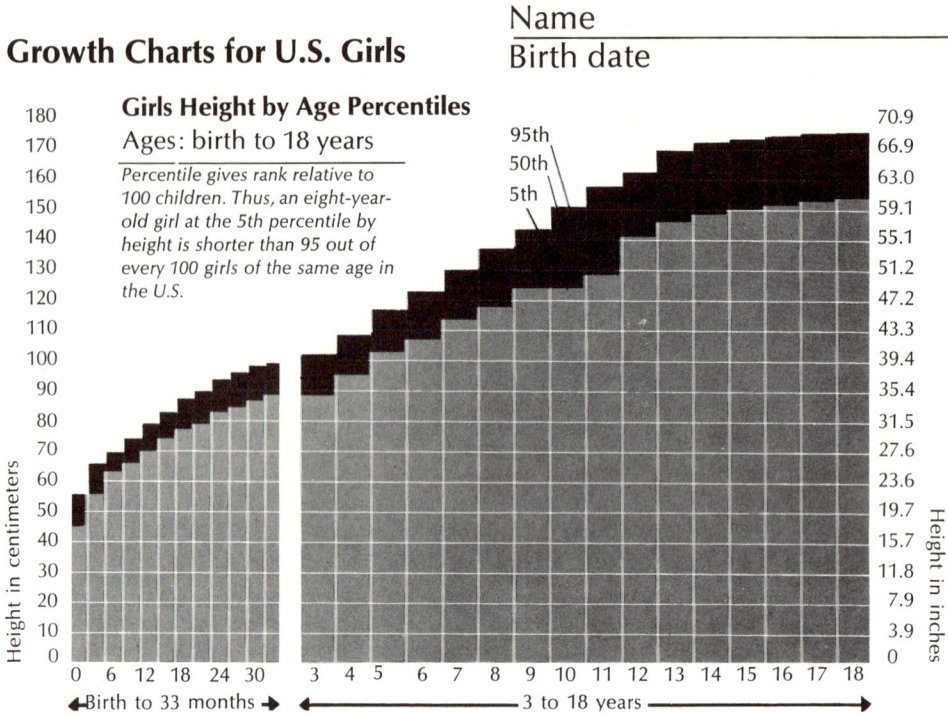

Girls Height by Age Percentiles

Ages: birth to 18 years

Percentile gives rank relative to 100 children. Thus, an eight-year-old girl at the 5th percentile by height is shorter than 95 out of every 100 girls of the same age in the U.S.

Height in centimeters

Height in inches

95th
50th
5th

0 6 12 18 24 30 ◄Birth to 33 months➤ 3 4 5 6 7 8 9 10 11 12 13 14 15 16 17 18 ◄───── 3 to 18 years ─────➤

Fig. 4-3

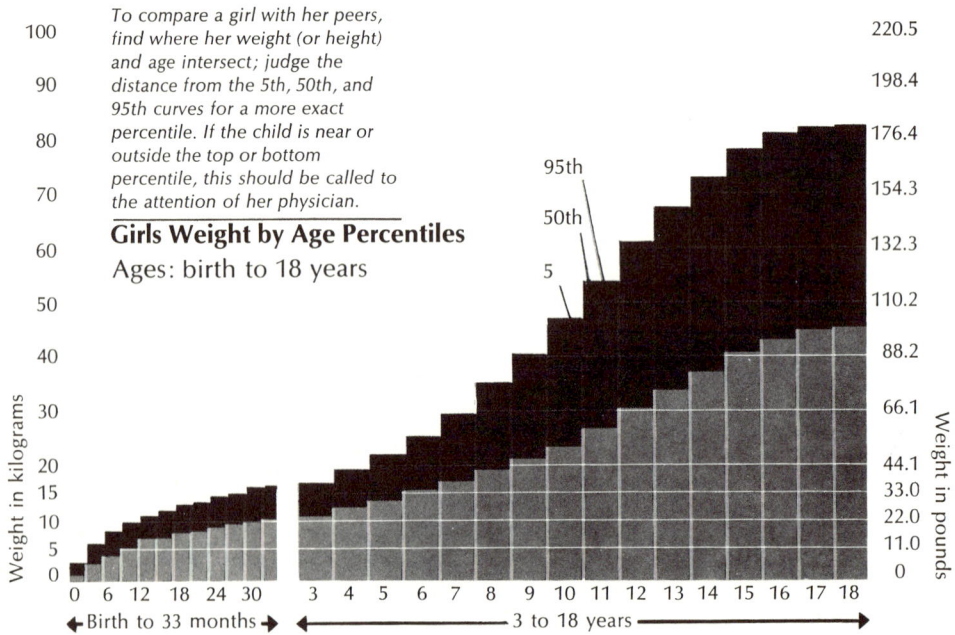

To compare a girl with her peers, find where her weight (or height) and age intersect; judge the distance from the 5th, 50th, and 95th curves for a more exact percentile. If the child is near or outside the top or bottom percentile, this should be called to the attention of her physician.

Girls Weight by Age Percentiles

Ages: birth to 18 years

Weight in kilograms

Weight in pounds

95th
50th
5

0 6 12 18 24 30 ◄Birth to 33 months➤ 3 4 5 6 7 8 9 10 11 12 13 14 15 16 17 18 ◄───── 3 to 18 years ─────➤

Fig. 4-4

Growth Charts for U.S. Boys

Name _____

Birth date _____

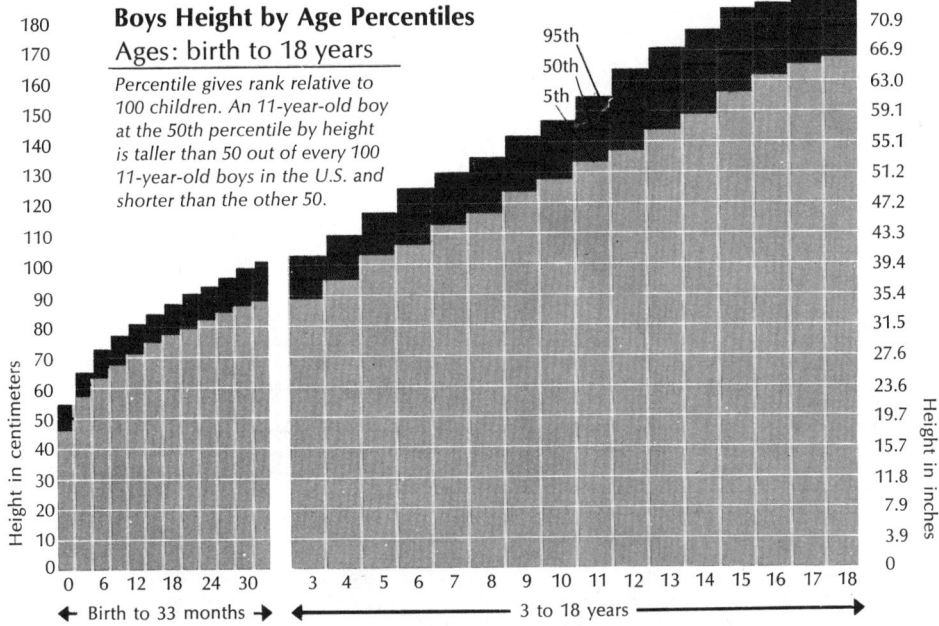

Boys Height by Age Percentiles

Ages: birth to 18 years

Percentile gives rank relative to 100 children. An 11-year-old boy at the 50th percentile by height is taller than 50 out of every 100 11-year-old boys in the U.S. and shorter than the other 50.

Height in centimeters

Height in inches

← Birth to 33 months →

3 to 18 years

Fig. 4-5

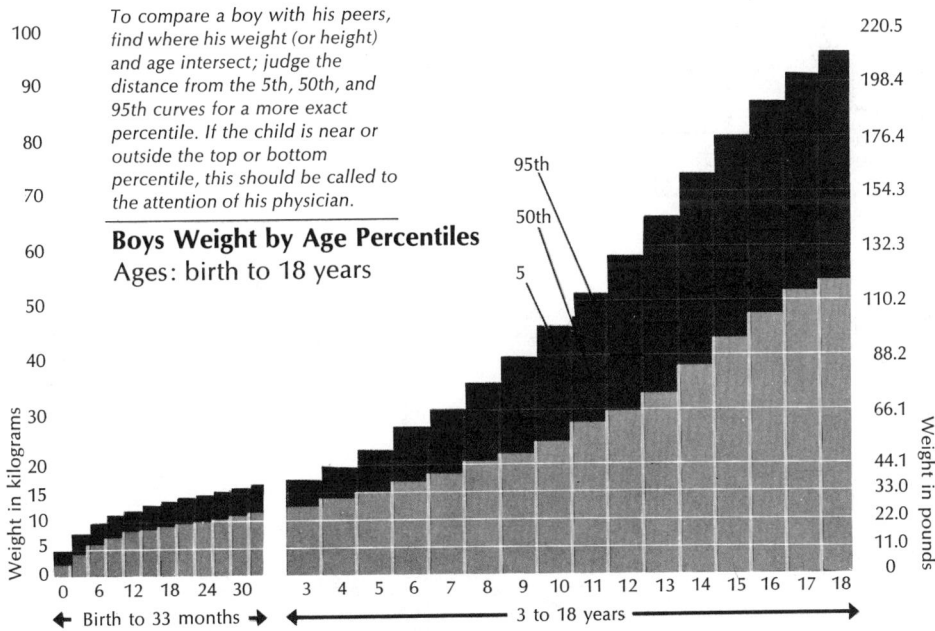

To compare a boy with his peers, find where his weight (or height) and age intersect; judge the distance from the 5th, 50th, and 95th curves for a more exact percentile. If the child is near or outside the top or bottom percentile, this should be called to the attention of his physician.

Boys Weight by Age Percentiles

Ages: birth to 18 years

Weight in kilograms

Weight in pounds

← Birth to 33 months →

3 to 18 years

Fig. 4-6

Girls from birth to 36 months

Head circumference for age

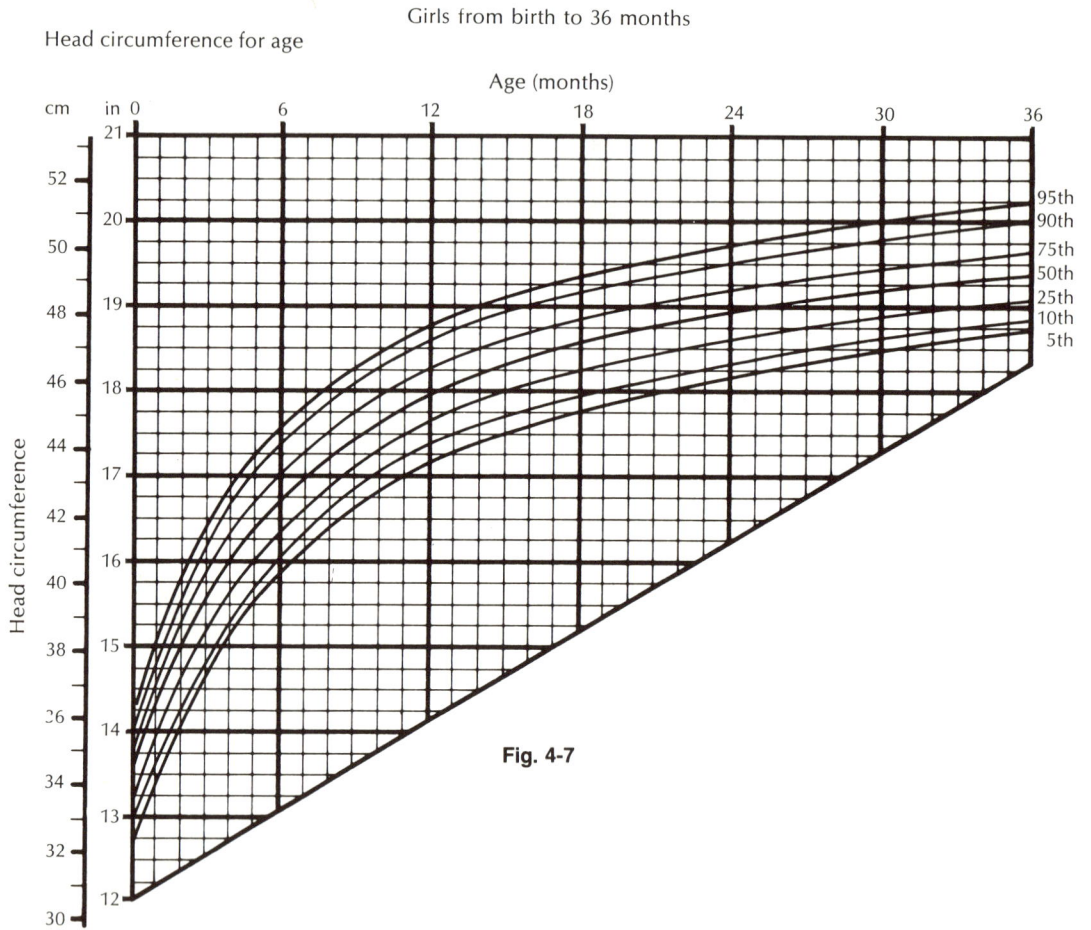

Fig. 4-7

Boys from birth to 36 months

Head circumference for age

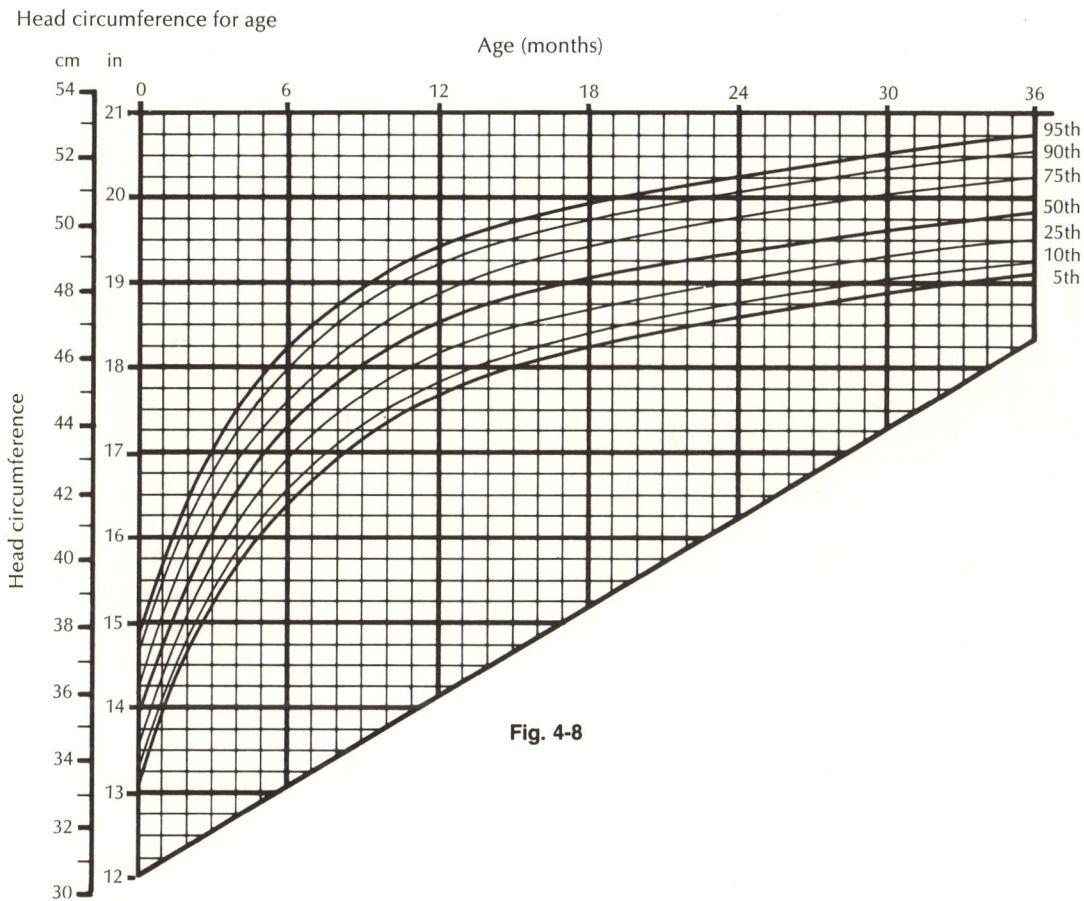

Fig. 4-8

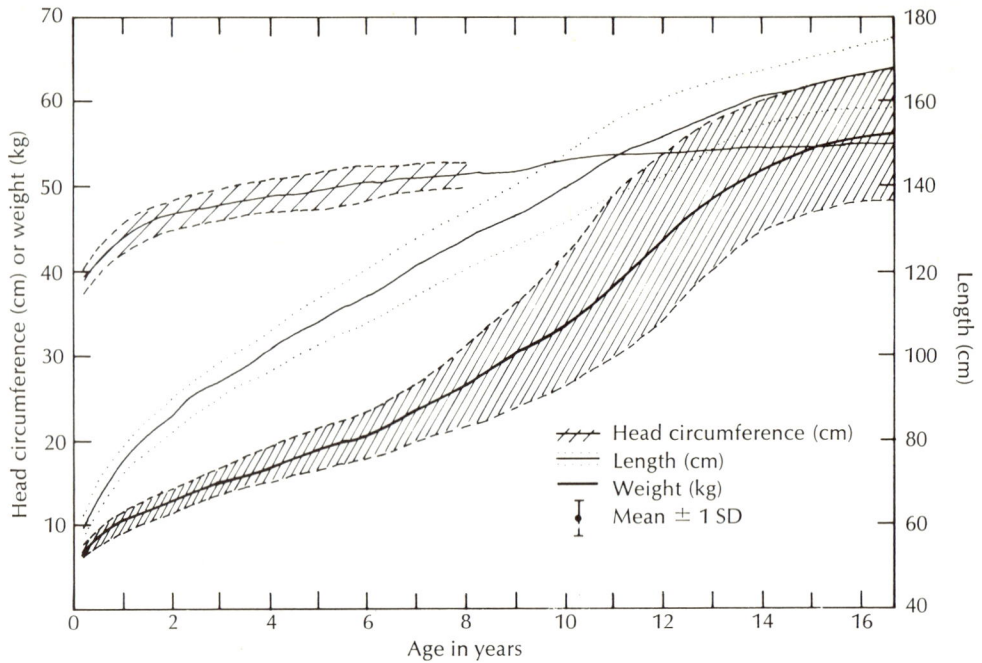

Fig. 4-9. Physical growth of black girls. (Derived from measurements obtained from 2,632 well children from low-income families in Washington, D.C. Abstracted from Verghese, K. P., Scott, R. B., Teixeira, G., and Ferguson, A. D.: Pediatrics **44**:243, 1969. Graphs were prepared from those of Freedmen's Hospital, Department of Pediatrics, Washington, D.C. Reprinted by permission of Roland B. Scott, M.D., Howard University College of Medicine, Washington, D.C.)

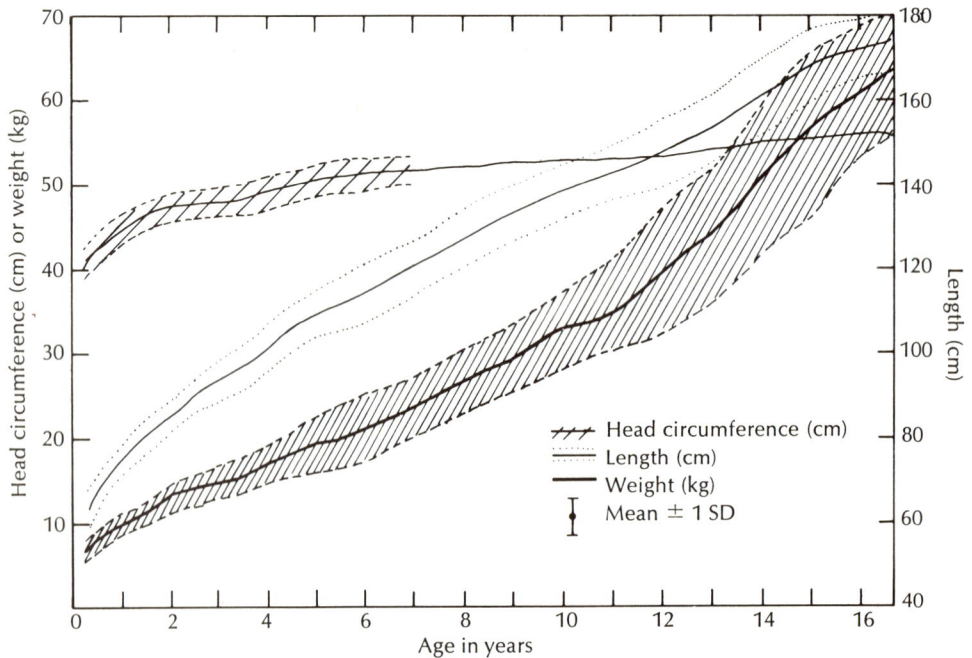

Fig. 4-10. Physical growth of black boys. (Derived from measurements obtained from 2,632 well children from low-income families in Washington, D.C. Abstracted from Verghese, K. P., Scott, R. B., Teixeira, G., and Ferguson, A. D.: Pediatrics **44**:243, 1969. Graphs were prepared from those of Freedmen's Hospital, Department of Pediatrics, Washington, D.C. Reprinted by permission of Roland B. Scott, M.D., Howard University College of Medicine, Washington, D.C.)

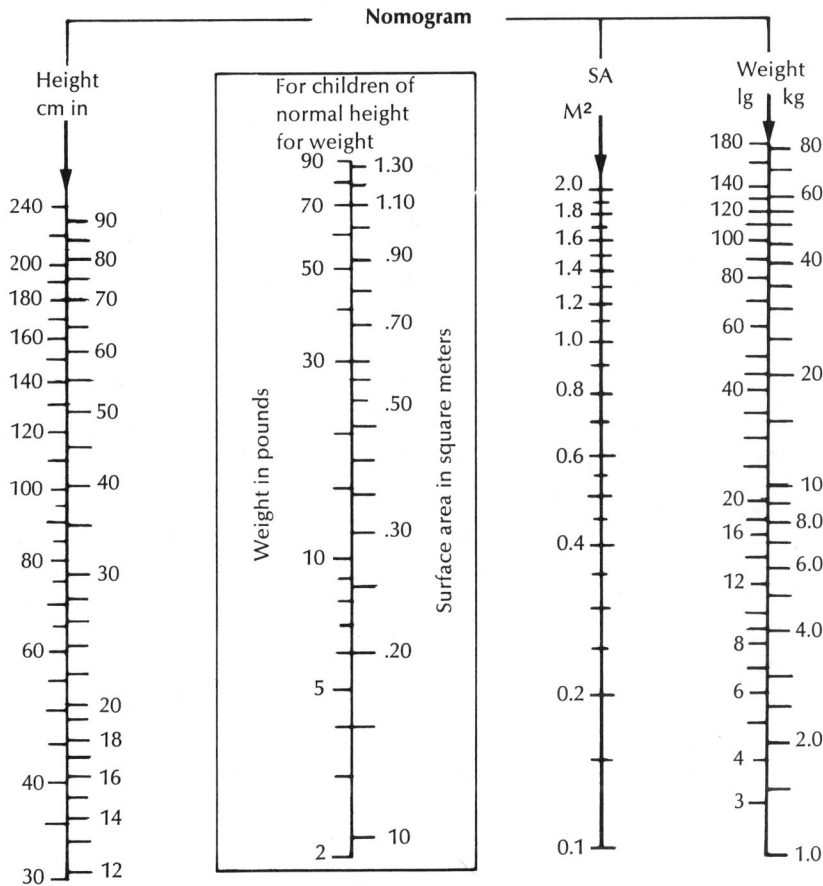

Fig. 4-11. West nomogram (for estimation of surface areas). The surface area is indicated where a straight line connecting the height and weight intersects the surface area (SA) column or, if the patient is roughly of normal proportion, from the weight alone (enclosed area). (Nomogram modified from data of E. Boyd by C. D. West. From Shirkey, H. C.: Drug therapy. In Nelson, W. E., Vaughan, V. C. III, and McKay, R. J., editors: Textbook of pediatrics, ed. 9, Philadelphia, 1969, W. B. Saunders Co.)

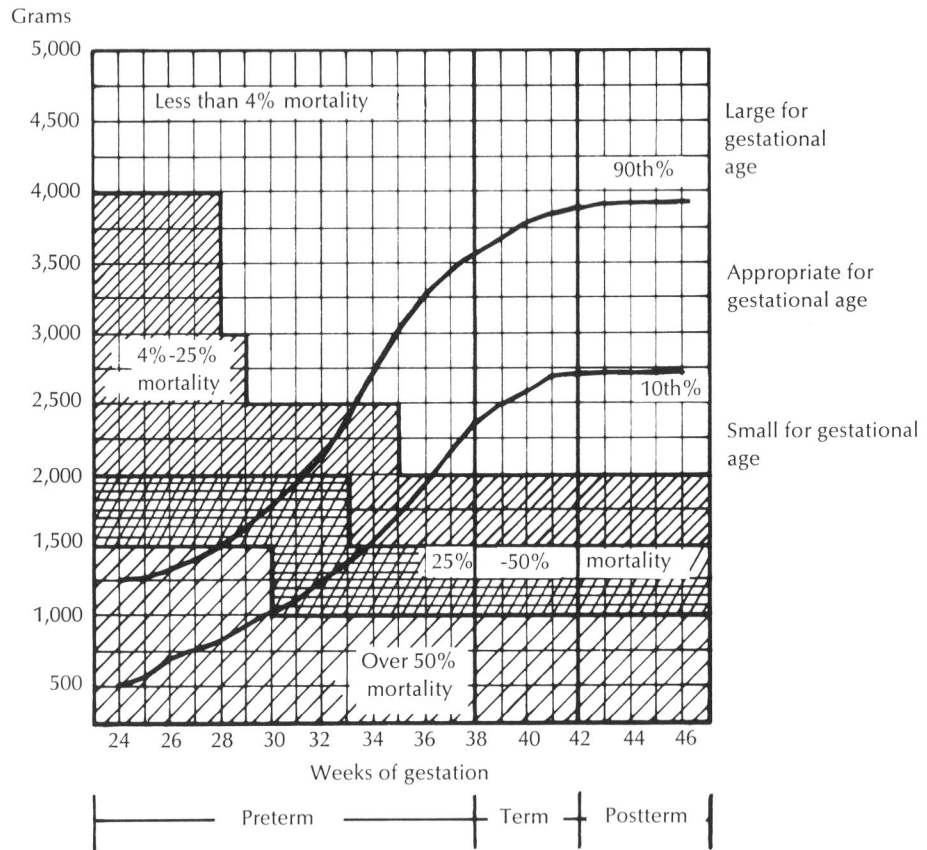

Fig. 4-12. Classification of newborns by birth weight and gestational age. (From Chinn, P.: Child health maintenance; concepts in family-centered care, ed. 2, St. Louis, 1979, The C. V. Mosby Co. After Battaglia, F. C., and Lubchenco, L. O.: J. Pediatr. **71:**161, 1967.)

Table 4-1. Chest circumference, boys and girls, birth to 5 years, in centimeters*

Percentile (boys)			Chest circumference	Percentile (girls)		
10	50	90		10	50	90
30.6	33.2	35.7	Birth	30.8	32.9	35.0
38.3	40.6	42.9	3 months	37.6	39.8	42.0
41.6	43.7	46.3	6 months	40.6	43.0	45.4
43.7	46.0	48.9	9 months	42.7	45.4	47.9
45.1	47.6	50.7	12 months	44.2	57.0	49.5
46.1	48.6	51.7	15 months	45.1	47.9	50.5
47.0	49.5	52.6	18 months	46.0	48.8	51.4
48.4	50.8	53.9	2 years	47.4	50.1	53.0
49.3	51.7	54.9	2½ years	48.4	51.2	54.3
49.9	52.4	55.8	3 years	49.3	51.9	55.1
50.5	53.1	56.6	3½ years	50.1	52.5	55.8
51.1	53.7	57.2	4 years	50.7	53.1	56.4
51.7	54.4	58.0	4½ years	51.3	53.7	57.3
52.3	55.0	58.8	5 years	51.7	54.2	57.9

*From Nelson, W. E., Vaughan, V. C. III, and McKay, R. J., editors: Textbook of pediatrics, ed. 9, Philadelphia, 1969, W. B. Saunders Co. From Studies of Child Health and Development, Department of Maternal and Child Health, Harvard School of Public Health.

Table 4-2. Chest circumference, boys and girls, 5 to 18 years, in centimeters*

Percentile (boys)			Chest circumference	Percentile (girls)		
10	50	90		10	50	90
51.6	54.5	57.5	5 years	50.2	52.9	56.5
52.4	55.3	58.5	5½ years	50.9	53.7	57.4
53.2	56.1	59.5	6 years	51.5	54.5	58.2
54.1	57.0	60.6	6½ years	52.2	55.3	59.2
54.9	57.8	61.6	7 years	52.8	56.1	60.1
55.8	58.8	62.9	7½ years	53.5	57.0	61.2
56.7	59.8	64.1	8 years	54.2	57.8	62.3
57.6	60.8	65.4	8½ years	54.9	58.7	63.5
58.4	61.8	66.7	9 years	55.5	59.6	64.7
59.3	62.9	68.1	9½ years	56.2	60.5	66.1
60.1	63.9	69.4	10 years	56.9	61.4	67.4
60.9	64.9	70.7	10½ years	57.8	62.8	69.0
61.7	65.9	71.9	11 years	58.6	64.2	70.5
62.5	66.9	73.1	11½ years	59.6	65.5	72.2
63.3	67.8	74.2	12 years	60.6	66.7	73.8
64.2	69.1	75.8	12½ years	61.8	67.7	75.3
65.0	70.3	77.4	13 years	62.9	68.6	76.7
66.3	72.4	79.4	13½ years	63.8	69.3	77.7
67.6	74.5	81.4	14 years	64.6	69.9	78.6
69.4	76.3	83.1	14½ years	65.1	70.4	79.2
71.1	78.0	84.8	15 years	65.5	70.9	79.8
72.8	79.4	86.3	15½ years	65.8	71.3	80.2
74.4	80.7	87.8	16 years	66.1	71.6	80.5
75.4	81.6	88.8	16½ years	66.3	71.9	80.7
76.4	82.5	89.7	17 years	66.4	72.1	80.9
77.0	83.0	90.2	17½ years	66.5	72.2	81.0
77.5	83.4	90.7	18 years	66.6	72.3	81.1

*From Nelson, W. E., Vaughan, V. C. III, and McKay, R. J., editors: Textbook of pediatrics, ed. 9, Philadelphia, 1969, W. B. Saunders Co. From Studies of Child Health and Development, Department of Maternal and Child Health, Harvard School of Public Health.

Table 4-3. Chest circumference for black children, in centimeters*

| | Chest circumference | | | |
| | Boys | | Girls | |
Age	Mean	SD	Mean	SD
3 months	38.2	3.3	38.1	1.8
6 months	41.7	1.9	40.2	2.4
9 months	42.7	2.5	41.7	2.8
12 months	43.7	2.4	43.6	1.8
15 months	44.4	2.3	44.2	2.8
18 months	46.2	2.9	45.3	2.6
21 months	47.4	2.4	46.4	2.9
24 months	48.6	3.4	47.0	3.3
2½ years	49.6	3.3	47.6	3.1
3 years	50.1	3.1	48.0	3.2
3½ years	50.7	3.4	48.4	3.4
4 years	50.8	4.0	48.9	3.1
4½ years	51.4	2.4	49.8	3.1
5 years	52.3	4.1	52.7	3.1
5½ years	54.3	3.6	53.5	3.8
6 years	56.5	3.8	54.7	3.8
7 years	58.5	3.6	56.0	3.2
8 years	60.8	3.0	58.2	4.6
9 years	62.9	3.4	60.4	6.4
10 years	64.5	4.5	62.0	5.2
11 years	66.5	3.7	64.4	7.0
12 years	70.3	5.4	66.1	4.0
13 years	73.6	5.7	67.6	6.1
14 years	76.8	5.9	68.0	4.2
15 years	80.7	5.6	68.6	5.3
16 years	83.8	4.5	70.2	3.8
17 years	85.6	6.3	70.8	9.5

For conversion: 1 inch = 2.54 cm

*Derived from measurements obtained from 2,632 well children from low-income families in Washington, D.C. Abstracted from Verghese, K. P., Scott, R. B., Teixeira, G., and Ferguson, A. D.: Studies in growth and development. XII. Physical growth of North American Negro children, Pediatrics **44**:243, Aug. 1969. Graphs prepared from those of Freedmen's Hospital, Department of Pediatrics, Washington, D.C.; reprinted by permission of Roland B. Scott, M.D., Howard University College of Medicine, Washington, D.C.

Table 4-4. Pulse rates for boys and girls up to 18 years*†

Age in years	Pulse rate per minute					
	Boys			Girls		
	No. of tests	Mean ± σ_m	SD	No. of tests	Mean ± σ_m	SD
0- 1	33	135 ± 3.1	18	56	126 ± 2.8	21
1- 2	82	105 ± 1.8	16	93	104 ± 1.8	17
2- 3	150	93 ± 1.0	12	177	93 ± 0.7	9
3- 4	157	87 ± 0.7	9	145	89 ± 0.7	9
4- 5	157	84 ± 0.7	8	137	84 ± 0.7	8
5- 6	150	79 ± 0.6	7	129	79 ± 0.6	7
6- 7	146	76 ± 0.6	8	122	77 ± 0.7	8
7- 8	140	75 ± 0.7	8	117	76 ± 0.8	8
8- 9	142	73 ± 0.7	9	114	73 ± 0.6	7
9-10	168	70 ± 0.6	7	106	70 ± 0.7	8
10-11	164	67 ± 0.6	7	98	69 ± 0.8	8
11-12	129	67 ± 0.6	7	84	69 ± 0.8	7
12-13	131	66 ± 0.6	7	72	69 ± 0.9	8
13-14	110	65 ± 0.8	8	68	68 ± 0.9	8
14-15	106	62 ± 0.7	7	57	66 ± 1.1	8
15-16	76	61 ± 0.9	8	47	65 ± 1.1	8
16-17	45	61 ± 0.9	6	30	66 ± 1.4	8
17-18	38	60 ± 1.4	8	20	65 ± 1.7	7

*Adapted from Iliff, A., and Lee, V. A.: Pulse rate, respiratory rate, and body temperature of children between 2 months and 18 years, Child Dev. **23**:237, 1952. By permission of the Society for Research in Child Development, Inc.
†Measurements were made following the basal metabolism determinations, and all those after 3 years were made in the morning.

Table 4-5. Respiratory rates for boys and girls up to 18 years*†

Age in years	Respiratory rate per minute					
	Boys			Girls		
	No. of tests	Mean ± σ_m	SD	No. of tests	Mean ± σ_m	SD
0- 1	38	31 ± 1.3	8	55	30 ± 0.8	6
1- 2	69	26 ± 0.5	4	79	27 ± 0.5	4
2- 3	118	25 ± 0.4	4	134	25 ± 0.3	3
3- 4	131	24 ± 0.2	3	119	24 ± 0.2	3
4- 5	122	23 ± 0.2	2	113	22 ± 0.2	2
5- 6	110	22 ± 0.2	2	100	21 ± 0.2	2
6- 7	128	21 ± 0.2	3	97	21 ± 0.3	3
7- 8	119	20 ± 0.2	3	97	20 ± 0.2	2
8- 9	113	20 ± 0.2	2	101	20 ± 0.2	2
9-10	141	19 ± 0.2	2	98	19 ± 0.2	2
10-11	141	19 ± 0.2	2	90	19 ± 0.2	2
11-12	123	19 ± 0.2	3	82	19 ± 0.3	3
12-13	131	19 ± 0.2	3	72	19 ± 0.3	2
13-14	110	19 ± 0.2	2	68	18 ± 0.3	2
14-15	106	18 ± 0.2	2	57	18 ± 0.4	3
15-16	76	17 ± 0.3	3	47	18 ± 0.4	3
16-17	45	17 ± 0.4	2	30	17 ± 0.5	3
17-18	38	16 ± 0.5	3	20	17 ± 0.7	3

*Adapted from Iliff, A., and Lee, V. A.: Pulse rate, respiratory rate, and body temperature of children between 2 months and 18 years, Child Dev. **23**:237, 1952. By permission of the Society for Research in Child Development, Inc.
†Measurements were made at the time of the basal metabolism determinations, and all those after 3 years were made in the morning.

Table 4-6. Body temperatures for boys and girls up to 18 years*†

| Age in years | Body temperature (°F) | | | | | |
| | Boys | | | Girls | | |
	No. of tests	Mean $\pm \sigma_m$	SD	No. of tests	Mean $\pm \sigma_m$	SD
0- 1	38	R 99.1 ± 0.12	0.7	57	R 99.1 ± 0.05	0.4
1- 2	86	R 99.1 ± 0.05	0.5	92	R 98.9 ± 0.05	0.5
2- 3	145	R 99.0 ± 0.03	0.4	167	R 98.8 ± 0.03	0.4
3- 4	96	R 98.9 ± 0.04	0.4	96	R 98.8 ± 0.04	0.4
3- 4	59	98.7 ± 0.06	0.5	45	98.7 ± 0.08	0.5
4- 5	116	98.6 ± 0.04	0.5	98	98.5 ± 0.06	0.5
5- 6	141	98.5 ± 0.04	0.4	121	98.5 ± 0.04	0.4
6- 7	144	98.4 ± 0.04	0.4	120	98.5 ± 0.04	0.4
7- 8	141	98.3 ± 0.04	0.4	117	98.4 ± 0.04	0.4
8- 9	142	98.3 ± 0.04	0.4	113	98.3 ± 0.03	0.4
9-10	167	98.1 ± 0.04	0.5	106	98.2 ± 0.04	0.4
10-11	163	98.0 ± 0.04	0.5	98	98.1 ± 0.04	0.4
11-12	129	98.0 ± 0.03	0.4	84	98.0 ± 0.05	0.5
12-13	131	97.8 ± 0.04	0.4	71	97.9 ± 0.05	0.4
13-14	110	97.7 ± 0.04	0.4	68	97.9 ± 0.06	0.5
14-15	106	97.6 ± 0.04	0.4	57	97.9 ± 0.08	0.6
15-16	76	97.4 ± 0.05	0.4	47	97.9 ± 0.06	0.4
16-17	45	97.3 ± 0.07	0.5	30	97.8 ± 0.09	0.5
17-18	38	97.2 ± 0.06	0.4	20	97.9 ± 0.12	0.5

*Adapted from Iliff, A., and Lee, V. A.: Pulse rate, respiratory rate, and body temperature of children between 2 months and 18 years, Child Dev. **23**:237, 1952. By permission of the Society for Research in Child Development, Inc.
†Measurements were made following the basal metabolism determinations, and all those after 3 years were made in the morning. Temperatures measured rectally are indicated by the letter "R"; other temperatures were taken orally.

Table 4-7. Normal blood pressure at various ages*

Ages	Mean systolic ± 2 SD	Mean diastolic ± 2 SD
Newborn	80 ± 16	46 ± 16
6-12 months	89 ± 29	60 ± 10
1 year	96 ± 30	66 ± 25
2 years	99 ± 25	64 ± 25
3 years	100 ± 25	67 ± 23
4 years	99 ± 20	65 ± 20
5-6 years	94 ± 14	55 ± 9
6-7 years	100 ± 15	56 ± 9
7-8 years	102 ± 15	56 ± 8
8-9 years	105 ± 16	57 ± 9
9-10 years	107 ± 16	57 ± 9
10-11 years	111 ± 17	58 ± 10
11-12 years	113 ± 18	59 ± 10
12-13 years	115 ± 19	59 ± 10
13-14 years	118 ± 19	60 ± 10

*From Haggerty, R. J., Maroney, M. W., and Nadas, A. S.: Essential hypertension in infancy and childhood, Am. J. Dis. Child. **92**:535, 1956. Copyright 1956, American Medical Association.

Table 4-8. Normal values for hematocrit and hemoglobin*

Hematocrit

Birth	44-64%
14-90 days	35-49%
6 months-1 year	30-40%
4-10 years	31-43%

Hemoglobin

Day 1	19 (14-24) g/100 ml
Day 2	19 (15-23) g/100 ml
Day 6	18 (13-23) g/100 ml
2 weeks	16.5 (15-20) g/100 ml
1 month	14 (11-17) g/100 ml
2 months	12 (11-14) g/100 ml
3 months	11 (10-13) g/100 ml
6 months	11.5 (10.5-14.5) g/100 ml
1 year	12 (11-15) g/100 ml
2 years	13 (12-15) g/100 ml
5 years	13.5 (12.5-15) g/100 ml
8-13 years	14 (13-15.5) g/100 ml

*From Kempe, C. H., Silver, H. K., and O'Brien, D.: Current pediatric diagnosis and treatment, ed. 2, Los Altos, Calif., 1972, Lange Medical Publications, p. 978.

NORMAL VALUES FOR LABORATORY TESTING OF BLOOD AND URINE

With the expanded responsibilities of health care professionals in providing primary care in a clinical setting, there is a greater demand for increased skills in certain laboratory procedures. Some procedures are simple, and a health aide may be trained to do them efficiently and accurately. Other techniques are best done in a laboratory by personnel who have been given expert training and where procedures are standardized. The type of procedure to be done will depend on several factors, including the ability and training of the personnel, the availability of laboratory resources, and the urgency to have laboratory information about the patient.

When laboratory procedures are provided, several principles should be kept in mind. First, the procedures must be standardized. Instruments should be maintained so that the information they provide is accurate. Each person involved in providing laboratory information should use consistent techniques that are frequently tested for reliability. Second, no procedures should be attempted by personnel when resources exist that can provide the same information with greater accuracy. Third, no procedure should be attempted when personnel are untrained or facilities are inadequate to provide accurate information.

There are several procedures that will add greatly to the information about the child during the assessment process.

1. *Hematocrit.* An assessment is not considered complete without information regarding the child's hematologic status (Table 4-8). This is a simple procedure, but it demands attention to detail to provide accurate information. The results of the hematocrit may be used for diet counseling or for referral when symptoms of anemia exist.

2. *Hemoglobin.* The hematocrit determination is done more frequently than determination of hemoglobin because the procedure is more simple and accurate (Table 4-8). Simple procedures are available for determination of hemoglobin, but the accuracy of procedures that require only the use of reagents without standardization is open to question.

3. *Urinalysis.* For most assessments a simple screening of the urine for absence of sugar, ketone bodies, and proteins by the use of test tapes is adequate. In addition, it is ideal to test the urine for evidence of bacteria. This may also be done with some degree of reliability by a test tape procedure. If there is evidence of bacteria, a urine culture may then be done in a laboratory, where the organism may be identified with great reliability.

4. *Throat culture.* It is not uncommon for a child to have group A beta hemolytic streptococci in the throat and remain asymptomatic. During the winter months and early spring it is not uncommon to isolate this organism in the throat during a routine examination, especially in regions of the country where the organism is most prevalent. Therefore, it is good practice to make this a common part of the assessment, especially in the school-age child. A throat culture is mandatory in a symptomatic child. There is no accurate way to determine the presence of the group A beta hemolytic streptococci other than by culture. It is not recommended that the practitioner attempt to grow the organism in a clinical setting. Generally, a regional laboratory has the equipment to accurately identify the organism. In many states a culture pac may be obtained from the state laboratory at minimal or no cost; this allows the exudate obtained from a throat swab to be mailed to the laboratory for culture.

5. *Phenylketonuria.* A simple routine blood test is required in most states to screen for phenylketonuria (PKU). A negative value should be present.

There are several additional procedures that add greatly to the information about the patient but which should not be attempted until adequate training has been completed. These procedures include the following.

1. *Blood smear.* This procedure requires a great deal of skill and training. Information obtained from a blood smear includes:
   a. Size, shape, and color of abnormal forms of red blood cells.
   b. Differential.

The normal values for a blood smear are:
   a. Normocytic/normochromic.
   b. Myeloid band, 7%; polymorphonuclear

leukocytes, 60%; eosinophils, 4%; basophils, 0.5% to 1% (lymphocytes, 25%; monocytes, 7%).*

2. *White blood cells, red blood cells.* Techniques for using the hemocytometer require considerable skill and patience and do not equal the electronic methods that are institutionally available.

The normal values are:

a. WBCs, 6,000 to 9,000/cu mm.

b. RBCs, 4.4 to 5.0 million/cu mm.

3. *Sickle cell anemia.* It would be ideal if every black child could be screened for the presence of sickle cell anemia or sickle cell trait. The procedure is relatively simple and fairly inexpensive. Reagents can be purchased from a laboratory supply house, and a sickle cell viewer, which is an additional (but a one-time) expense, may also be purchased. The test may be done on heparinized blood from a venous supply or from a finger or heel prick. Although there is an initial investment in material, reagents remain stable for as long as 1 year.

4. *Lead.* The urine may be screened for the presence of lead. This is a complex procedure and is most often done in a laboratory through the use of a spectrometer. It would be ideal if every child in an area that is known to have a risk of lead ingestion were to have this determination frequently.

---

*In children up to 7 years there may be more lymphocytes and fewer polymorphonuclear leukocytes. In bacterial infections, the WBC count is raised, and in viral infections the WBC count may be lowered, with an increased lymphocyte count. In parasitic infections eosinophils are increased.

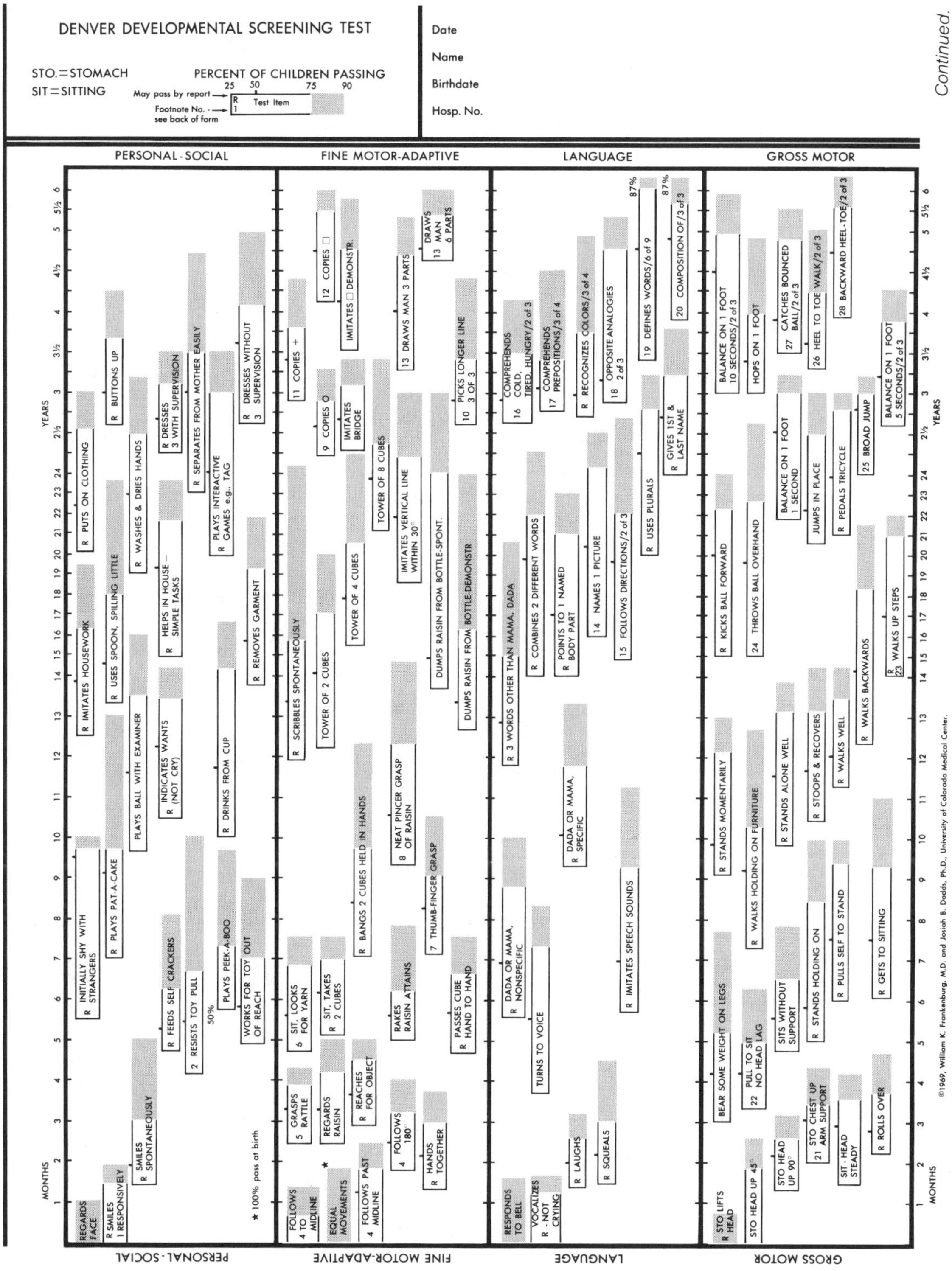

Fig. 4-13. Denver Developmental Screening Test. (Courtesy William K. Frankenburg, M.D., University of Colorado Medical Center, Denver, Colo.)

Continued.

1. Try to get child to smile by smiling, talking or waving to him. Do not touch him.
2. When child is playing with toy, pull it away from him. Pass if he resists.
3. Child does not have to be able to tie shoes or button in the back.
4. Move yarn slowly in an arc from one side to the other, about 6" above child's face.
   Pass if eyes follow 90° to midline. (Past midline; 180°)
5. Pass if child grasps rattle when it is touched to the backs or tips of fingers.
6. Pass if child continues to look where yarn disappeared or tries to see where it went. Yarn
   should be dropped quickly from sight from tester's hand without arm movement.
7. Pass if child picks up raisin with any part of thumb and a finger.
8. Pass if child picks up raisin with the ends of thumb and index finger using an over hand
   approach.

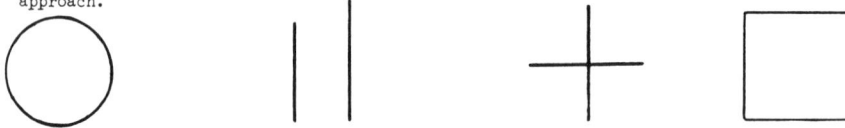

9. Pass any enclosed form. Fail continuous round motions.
10. Which line is longer? (Not bigger.) Turn paper upside down and repeat. (3/3 or 5/6)
11. Pass any crossing lines.
12. Have child copy first. If failed, demonstrate

When giving items 9, 11 and 12, do not name the forms. Do not demonstrate 9 and 11.

13. When scoring, each pair (2 arms, 2 legs, etc.) counts as one part.
14. Point to picture and have child name it. (No credit is given for sounds only.)

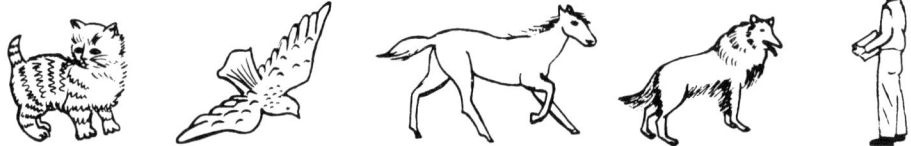

15. Tell child to: Give block to Mommie; put block on table; put block on floor. Pass 2 of 3.
    (Do not help child by pointing, moving head or eyes.)
16. Ask child: What do you do when you are cold? ..hungry? ..tired? Pass 2 of 3.
17. Tell child to: Put block on table; under table; in front of chair, behind chair.
    Pass 3 of 4. (Do not help child by pointing, moving head or eyes.)
18. Ask child: If fire is hot, ice is ?; Mother is a woman, Dad is a ?; a horse is big, a
    mouse is ?. Pass 2 of 3.
19. Ask child: What is a ball? ..lake? ..desk? ..house? ..banana? ..curtain? ..ceiling?
    ..hedge? ..pavement? Pass if defined in terms of use, shape, what it is made of or general
    category (such as banana is fruit, not just yellow). Pass 6 of 9.
20. Ask child: What is a spoon made of? ..a shoe made of? ..a door made of? (No other objects
    may be substituted.) Pass 3 of 3.
21. When placed on stomach, child lifts chest off table with support of forearms and/or hands.
22. When child is on back, grasp his hands and pull him to sitting. Pass if head does not hang back.
23. Child may use wall or rail only, not person. May not crawl.
24. Child must throw ball overhand 3 feet to within arm's reach of tester.
25. Child must perform standing broad jump over width of test sheet. (8-1/2 inches)
26. Tell child to walk forward,   heel within 1 inch of toe.
    Tester may demonstrate. Child must walk 4 consecutive steps, 2 out of 3 trials.
27. Bounce ball to child who should stand 3 feet away from tester. Child must catch ball with
    hands, not arms, 2 out of 3 trials.
28. Tell child to walk backward,   toe within 1 inch of heel.
    Tester may demonstrate. Child must walk 4 consecutive steps, 2 out of 3 trials.

DATE AND BEHAVIORAL OBSERVATIONS (how child feels at time of test, relation to tester, attention
span, verbal behavior, self-confidence, etc,):

Fig. 4-13, cont'd. Denver Developmental Screening Test.

DEVELOPMENT OF SPEECH, LANGUAGE, AND HEARING

Table 4-9. Landmarks of speech, language, and hearing ability*

Chronologic age	Receptive language	Expressive language	Related hearing ability
3 months			Is startled by loud sounds and soothed by mother's voice. Lateral turning to the side of sound; turning in general direction, but not looking directly at sound source.
6 months	Responds by raising arms when mother says come here and reaches toward the child; responds appropriately to friendly or angry voices; moves or looks toward family member when named.	Repeats self-produced sounds; imitates sounds; vocalizes to persons; uses 12 different phonemes.	Turns eyes and head to search for location of sound, but does not necessarily find the sound source on the first attempt. Responds to mother's voice and own name, imitates own noises, and enjoys sound-making toys.
8 months			Turns eyes and head in a sweeping motion to the sound source. Locates sound source.
10 months			Looks directly, promptly, and predictably to the sound source. Responds to own name, telephone ringing, and someone's voice.
12 months	Up to 10 words, such as no, bye-bye, pat-a-cake, hot, own name; one simple direction, such as sit down or give it to me; these commands are usually accompanied by gesture.	Up to 3 words besides mama and dada; may say such words as bye-bye, hi, baby, kitty, and puppy; uses up to 18 different phonemes.	Begins to show voluntary control over responses to sound; may or may not respond, or may delay response. This selective response should not be interpreted as a hearing loss so long as it is intermittent and of recent origin. This might be representative of beginning of listening refinement.
18 months	Up to 50 words; recognizes between 6 and 12 objects by name, such as dog, cat, bottle, ball; identifies 3 body parts, such as eyes, nose, mouth; understands the concept "now," simple commands unaccompanied by gesture, such as give me the doll, open your mouth, stick out your tongue.	Up to 20 words and 21 different phonemes; jargon and echolalia are present; uses names of familiar objects and 1-word sentences such as go or eat; uses gestures; uses words such as no, mine, eat, good, bad, hot, cold, and expressions such as oh-oh, what's that, all gone; the use of words may be quite inconsistent; 25% of speech is intelligible.	Has begun to develop gross discrimination by learning to distinguish between highly dissimilar noises such as doorbell and train, barking dog and auto horn, or mother's and father's voice.

*Adapted from Weiss, C. E., and Lillywhite, H. S.: Communicative disorders, St. Louis, 1976, The C. V. Mosby Co., pp. 51, 54-58, 65-66.

Continued.

Table 4-9. Landmarks of speech, language, and hearing ability—cont'd

Chronologic age	Receptive language	Expressive language	Related hearing ability
24 months	Up to 1,200 words; in, on, under; identifies dog, ball, engine, bed, doll, scissors, hair, mouth, feet, nose, cup, spoon, car, key; distinguishes between one and many, and formulates negative judgment—a knife is not a fork; understands the concept "soon," simple stories; follows simple directions; is beginning to make distinctions between you and me.	Up to 270 words and 25 different phonemes; jargon and echolalia almost gone; averages 75 words per hour during free play; talks in words, phrases, and 2- to 3-word sentences; averages 2 words per response; first pronouns appear, such as I, me, mine, it, who, that; adjectives and adverbs are just beginning to appear; names objects and common pictures; enjoys Mother Goose; refers to self by name, such as Bobby go bye-bye; uses phrases such as I want, go bye-bye, want cookie, ball all gone; 60% of speech is intelligible.	Refinement of gross discriminative skills.
30 months	Up to 2,400 words; identifies action in pictures and objects by use; carries out 1- and 2-part commands such as pick up your shoe and give it to mommy; knows what we drink out of, what goes on our feet, what we can buy candy with; understands plurals, questions, difference between boy and girl, the concept "one," up, down, run, walk, throw, fast, more, my.	Up to 425 words and 27 phonemes; jargon and echolalia no longer exist; averages 140 words per hour; names words such as chair, can, box, key, door; repeats 2 digits from memory; average sentence length is about 2½ words; uses more adjectives and adverbs; demands repetition from others, such as do it again; almost always announces intentions before acting; begins to ask questions of adults; 75% of speech is intelligible.	
36 months	Up to 3,600 words; understands both, two, not today, what we do when we are thirsty, hungry, sleepy, why we have stoves, wait, later, big, new, different, strong, today, another, and taking turns at play; carries out 2- and some 3-item commands such as give me the ball, pick up the doll, and sit down; identifies several colors, and is aware of past and future.	Up to 900 words in simple sentences averaging 3-4 words per sentence; averages 15,000 words per day and 170 words per hour; uses words such as when, time, today, not today, new, different, big, strong, surprise, secret; can repeat 3 digits, name 1 color, say name, give simple account of experiences, and tell stories that can be understood; begins to use more pronouns, adjectives, and adverbs; describes at least 1 element of a picture; is aware of past and future; uses commands such as you make it; also expressions such as I can't, I don't want to; verbalizes toilet needs, and expresses desire to take turns; communication includes criticisms, commands, requests, threats, questions, answers; 85% of speech is intelligible.	Starts to distinguish dissimilar speech sounds such as the difference between "ee" and "er," although there may be some difficulty with the concepts of "same" and "different."

Table 4-9. Landmarks of speech, language, and hearing ability—cont'd

Chronologic age	Receptive language	Expressive language	Related hearing ability
42 months	Up to 4,200 words; knows words such as what, where, how, funny, we, surprise, secret; knows number concepts to 2, how to answer questions accurately, such as do you have a dog, which is the girl, what toys do you have.	Up to 1,200 words in mostly complete sentences averaging 4-5 words per sentence; uses all 50 phonemes; 7% of sentences are compound or complex; averages 203 words per hour; rate of speech is faster; relates experiences, and tells about activities in sequential order; uses words such as what, where, how, see, little, funny, they, we, he, she, several; can say a nursery rhyme; asks permission; 95% of speech is intelligible.	
48 months	Up to 5,600 words; carries out 3-item commands consistently; knows why we have houses, books, umbrella, key; knows nearly all the colors, words such as somebody, anybody, even, almost, now, something, like, bigger, too, full name, 1 or 2 songs, number concepts to 4; understands most preschool stories; can complete opposite analogies such as brother is a boy, sister is a _____; in daytime it is light, at night it is _____.	Up to 1,500 words in sentences averaging 5-6 words per sentence; averages 400 words per hour; counts to 3, repeats 4 digits, names 3 objects, and repeats 9-word sentences from memory; names the primary colors, some coins; relates fanciful tales; enjoys rhyming nonsense words and using exaggerations; demands reasons why and how; questioning is at a peak, up to 500 a day; passes judgment on own activity; can recite a poem from memory or sing a song; uses words such as even, almost, something, like, but; typical expressions might include I'm so tired, you almost hit me, now I'll make something else.	Begins to make fine discriminations among similar speech sounds such as the difference between "f" and "th" or "f" and "s." The child has matured enough to be tested with an audiometer. At this age formal hearing testing can usually be carried out. Not only has hearing developed to its optimum level, but listening has also become considerably refined.
54 months	Up to 6,500 words; knows what a house, window, chair, and dress are made of and what we do with our eyes and ears; understands differences in texture and composition, such as hard, soft, rough, smooth; begins to name or point to penny, nickel, dime; understands if, because, why, when.	Up to 1,800 words in sentences averaging 5-6 words; now averages only 230 words per hour—is satisfied with less verbalization; does little commanding or demanding; likes surprises; about 1 in 10 sentences is compound or complex, and only 8% of sentences are incomplete; can define 10 common words and count to 20; common expressions are I don't know, I said, tiny, funny, because; asks questions for information, and learns to manipulate and control persons and situations with language.	

Continued.

Table 4-9. Landmarks of speech, language, and hearing ability—cont'd

Chronologic age	Receptive language	Expressive language	Related hearing ability
60 months	Up to 9,600 words; knows number concepts to 5; knows and·names colors; defines words in terms of use, such as a horse is to ride; also defines wind, ball, hat, stove; understands words such as if, because, when; knows what the following are for: horse, fork, legs; begins to understand right and left.	Up to 2,200 words in sentences averaging 6 words; can define ball, hat, stove, policeman, wind, horse, fork; can count 5 objects and repeat 4 or 5 digits; definitions are in terms of use; can single out a word and ask its meaning; makes serious inquiries—what is this for, how does this work, who made those, what does it mean; language is now essentially complete in structure and form; uses all types of sentences, clauses, and parts of speech; reads by way of pictures, and prints simple words.	
66 months	Up to 13,500 words; knows number concepts to 7, right and left, most simple, compound, and complex sentences if not too long; knows functions of body parts—what are your eyes, ears, and so on for; understands dependent clauses such as when I open the door, put the cat out.	Up to 2,300 words; sentence length varies from 6-7 words; grammatical errors continue to decrease as sentences and vocabulary become more sophisticated.	
72 months	Up to 15,000 words; knows number concepts to 10, the meaning of morning, afternoon, night, summer, winter; can relate differences between objects, animals, and clothing; is beginning to answer a few similarities correctly, such in what way are_____ and_____alike.	Up to 2,500 words in sentences averaging 7 words; relates fanciful tales; recites numbers to 30; asks meaning of words; repeats 5 digits from memory; can complete analogies such as a table is made of wood and a window of _____, a bird flies and a fish _____, an inch is short and a mile is_____.	

Instructions: Have child repeat each word after you. Circle the underlined sounds that he pronounces correctly. Total correct sounds is the raw score. Use charts.

Name:
Hosp. No.:
Address:

Date:_____Child's Age:_____Examiner:_____Raw Score:_____

Percentile:_____Intelligibility:_____ _____Results:_____

1. table   6. zipper   11. sock   16. wagon   21. leaf
2. shirt   7. grapes   12. vacuum   17. gum   22. carrot
3. door   8. flag   13. yarn   18. house
4. trunk   9. thumb   14. mother   19. pencil
5. jumping   10. toothbrush   15. twinkle   20. fish

Intelligibility: (circle one)   1. Easy to understand
                                 2. Understandable 1/2 the time
                                 3. Not understandable
                                 4. Can't evaluate

Comments:

Date:_____Child's Age:_____Examiner:_____Raw Score:_____

Percentile:_____Intelligibility:_____Results:_____

1. table   6. zipper   11. sock   16. wagon   21. leaf
2. shirt   7. grapes   12. vacuum   17. gum   22. carrot
3. door   8. flag   13. yarn   18. house
4. trunk   9. thumb   14. mother   19. pencil
5. jumping   10. toothbrush   15. twinkle   20. fish

Intelligibility: (circle one)   1. Easy to understand
                                 2. Understandable 1/2 the time
                                 3. Not understandable
                                 4. Can't evaluate

Comments:

Continued.

Fig. 4-14. Denver articulation screening exam for children 2½ to 6 years of age.

To score DASE words: Note raw score for child's performance. Match raw score line (extreme left of chart) with column representing child's age (to the closest *previous* age group). Where raw score line and age column meet number in that square denotes percentile rank of child's performance when compared to other children that age. Percentiles above heavy line are *Abnormal* percentiles, below heavy line are *Normal*.

Percentile rank

Raw score	2.5 yr.	3.0	3.5	4.0	4.5	5.0	5.5	6 years
2	1							
3	2							
4	5							
5	9							
6	16							
7	23							
8	31	2						
9	37	4	1					
10	42	6	2					
11	48	7	4					
12	54	9	6	1	1			
13	58	12	9	2	3	1	1	
14	62	17	11	5	4	2	2	
15	68	23	15	9	5	3	2	
16	75	31	19	12	5	4	3	
17	79	38	25	15	6	6	4	
18	83	46	31	19	8	7	4	
19	86	51	38	24	10	9	5	1
20	89	58	45	30	12	11	7	3
21	92	65	52	36	15	15	9	4
22	94	72	58	43	18	19	12	5
23	96	77	63	50	22	24	15	7
24	97	82	70	58	29	29	20	15
25	99	87	78	66	36	34	26	17
26	99	91	84	75	46	43	34	24
27		94	89	82	57	54	44	34
28		96	94	88	70	68	59	47
29		98	98	94	84	84	77	68
30		100	100	100	100	100	100	100

To Score intelligibility:

		Normal	Abnormal
	2½ years	Understandable 1/2 time, or "easy"	Not understandable
	3 years and older	Easy to understand	Understandable 1/2 time Not understandable

Test Result: 1. *Normal* on DASE and Intelligibility = *Normal*
2. *Abnormal* on DASE and/or Intelligibility = *Abnormal*

*If abnormal on initial screening rescreen within 2 weeks. If abnormal again child should be referred for complete speech evaluation.

Fig. 4-14, cont'd. Denver articulation screening exam for children 2½ to 6 years of age.

VISUAL ASSESSMENT

Table 4-10. Landmarks of visual development*

Age	Characteristic development	Age	Characteristic development
Birth	Pupils react to light. Blink reflex in response to light stimulus. Corneal reflex in response to touch. Rudimentary fixation on objects with ability to follow to the midline.	28 to 44 weeks	Depth perception begins to develop. Displays interest in tiny objects. Tilts head backward to see upward. Exhibits smooth visual pursuit of objects and sound in the vertical and horizontal planes. Visual acuity exceeds 20/200.
2 to 4 weeks	Fixation ability advances; stares at light source. Follows to midline more reliably. Tear glands begin to function.	44 weeks to 12 months	Transverse diameter of the cornea is 12 mm, the adult size. Amblyopia may develop with lack of binocularity.
4 to 12 weeks	Convergence appears. Binocular fixation is established. Follows moving object with head and eye movements through 180°. Fascinated by bright colors and lights. Tear glands display response to emotion.		Fixates intently on facial expressions. Discriminates simple geometric forms Visual acuity 20/100. Full binocular vision developed.
12 to 20 weeks	Begins to inspect own hands. Accommodation begins to develop. Able to fixate on objects more than 3 feet distant. Foveal pit becomes distinguishable as macular development proceeds. Pigmentation of fundus not developed; appearance of fundus is pale. Visual acuity 20/200.	12 to 18 months	Able to identify forms. Associates with visual experiences. Displays an intent interest in pictures. Able to scribble on paper. Convergence becomes well established. Depth perception remains crude.
20 to 28 weeks	Able to rescue a dropped block. Hand-eye coordination is developing. Binocular fixation becomes fully developed. Ultimate color of iris is established. Discrimination between simple geometric forms is beginning to develop. Color preference for reds and yellows develops.	18 months to 2 years	Accommodation well developed. Visual acuity 20/40.
		2 to 3 years	Convergence smooth. Fixation on small objects or pictures should approach 50 seconds. Able to recall visual images. Visual acuity 20/30.
		3 years to 4 years	Able to copy geometric figures. Reading readiness is present. Lacrimal glands are fully developed.
		5 years	Minimal potential for amblyopia to develop. Color recognition is well established.
		6 years	Visual acuity approaches 20/20. Color shading may be differentiated. Astigmatism may develop at any point throughout life. Depth perception fully developed.

*Adapted from Whipple, D. V.: Dynamics of development; euthenic pediatrics, New York, 1966, McGraw-Hill Book Co.; Liebman, S. D., and Gellis, S. S.: The pediatrician's ophthalmology, St. Louis, 1966, The C. V. Mosby Co.; Keeney, A. H.: Development of vision. In Falkner, F., editor: Human development, Philadelphia, 1966, W. B. Saunders Co.

Table 4-11. Denver Eye Screening Test*†

Vision tests	First screening: date						Rescreening: date					
	Right eye			**Left eye**			**Right eye**			**Left eye**		
	Normal	Abnormal	Untestable	Normal	Abnormal	Untestable	Normal	Abnormal	Untestable	Normal	Abnormal	Untestable
1. "E" (3 years and above—3 to 5 trials)	3P	3F	U	3P	3F	U	3P	3F	U	3P	3F	U
2. Picture card ($2\frac{1}{2}$ to $2\frac{11}{12}$ yrs—3 to 5 trials)	3P	3F	U	3P	3F	U	3P	3F	U	3P	3F	U
3. Fixation (6 months to $2\frac{5}{12}$ yrs)	P	F	U	P	F	U	P	F	U	P	F	U
4. Squinting		Yes			Yes			Yes			Yes	

Tests for non-straight eyes	Normal	Abnormal	Untestable	Normal	Abnormal	Untestable
1. Do your child's eyes turn in or out, or are they ever not straight?	No	Yes		No	Yes	
2. Cover test	P	F		P	F	
3. Pupillary light reflex	P	F	U	P	F	U
	Date:			Date:		

Total test rating (both eyes)

	First screening	Rescreening
Normal (passed vision test plus no squint, plus passed ⅔ tests for nonstraight eyes)	Normal	Normal
Abnormal (abnormal on any vision test, squinting on 2 of 3 procedures for nonstraight eyes)	Abnormal	Abnormal
Untestable (untestable on any vision test or untestable on ⅔ tests for nonstraight eyes)	Untestable	Untestable
Future rescreening appointment for total test rating (abnormal or untestable)		

*From Barker, J., Goldstein, A., and Frankenburg, W. K.: Denver Eye Screening Test, 1972 edition, copyright 1972 by William K. Frankenburg.
†Manual and kit available from LADOCA Project and Publishing Foundation, Inc., East 51st Ave. and Lincoln Street, Denver, Colo. 80216.

Procedure and standardization for Snellen screening

Setup for screening

1. Hang the Snellen chart on a wall or large portable tackboard covered with white paper. Secure the chart to the board so that it does not swing. Use four rings of masking tape on the reverse corners of the chart to avoid defacing the chart.

2. Children ages 6 to 12 stand for the screening. Therefore, hang the chart so the 20- to 30-foot lines are at the level of the child's eyes. Older children will sit on a chair during the screening. This eliminates the necessity for moving the chart up and down.

3. Measure and place a piece of masking tape on the floor at a point 20 feet from the Snellen chart. Use a 20-foot tape to ensure accuracy. Fasten paper footprints to the floor with the *heels* edging the 20-foot line. When the child is seated, the back of the chair seat should be on the 20-foot line (at the heel of the footprints).

4. The light on the chart should be 10 to 30 foot-candles, and there should be no glare from the windows. Approximately 20 foot-candles is ideal. Control the light with blinds and drapes. Recheck periodically with a light meter.

5. Provide a clean eye cover card for each child; discard after use.

6. *If a child wears glasses, screen with glasses only.* When necessary, demonstrate proper care and cleaning of glasses (cleansing tissues). *Postpone the screening if a child does not have his or her glasses the day of the screening.* If the glasses are lost or broken, screen without glasses and make a note.

7. Two persons (may be volunteers) are needed to screen adequately.

Procedure

1. Glasses. If glasses have been prescribed previously, screen only with glasses. If the child doesn't have his or her glasses, screen without glasses and record under "Observations" the reason for not wearing them. When necessary, demonstrate the proper care and cleaning of glasses with cleansing tissue.

2. Instruct the child to keep both eyes open and not to press the occluder (cover card) against the eye. The edge should rest across the bridge of the nose.

3. Screen the right eye, then the left, and record in the same sequence. Record all information in the appropriate columns.

4. Use covers to expose one symbol or one line at a time.

5. When screening kindergarten children, expose one entire line and use a pointer stick to point to each symbol. After completing each line, cover that line and continue on to the next line using the same method.

6. If the child fails to read the symbols from left to right on a line, start the line over pointing right to left. When pointing to the symbols, be sure that the child is indicating the position of the symbol and is not reading ahead of the screener.

7. Have the child point with the entire arm and hand in the direction the legs of the "E" point. The occluder (cover card) volunteer starts the screening by saying "Show me which way the legs point on the chart."

8. To assist the volunteer at the chart and avoid distracting the child, the following signal system may be helpful. The volunteer at the chart shows the symbols one at a time and always begins with symbols on the 40-foot line, showing all four as the occluder (cover card) volunteer indicates that the child has demonstrated the different "E" positions by saying "Good," "Fine," "Right," or "Okay" (single words) after each symbol of each line. The last symbol on the line always receives the comment "Very good" (if the child passed the line by getting three out of four symbols correct) or "That's fine" (if he did not read three out of four symbols on any single line). Do not accumulate misses beyond one line. If the occluder volunteer says "Very good," the chart volunteer drops down one line to the 30-foot line and follows the same procedure as above. If the occluder volunteer says "That's fine," the chart volunteer moves to the top of the chart.

9. Begin at the 40-foot line and have the child read each symbol on every line below that. A child who reads three out of four symbols can see the line satisfactorily. Some lines have six symbols instead of four. In this case, the child should read four out of six.

10. If the child fails to read the 40-foot line, begin again, but at the top of the chart and move downward to find his or her level. Continue

RECORDING ACUITY

X	Unable to read 200 foot line	
200 foot line	Pupil must read all symbols	If pupil misses one or more symbols on
100 foot line	Pupil must read all symbols	these, record as line above
70 foot line	Pupil must read all symbols	
50 foot line	Pupil may miss one symbol	If pupil misses two or more symbols on
40 foot line	Pupil may miss one symbol	these, record as line above
30 foot line	Pupil may miss two symbols	If pupil misses three or more symbols
20 foot line	Pupil may miss two symbols	on these, record as line above

The pupil must read 3 out of 4 or 4 out of 6 symbols on a line correctly.

downward through the 20-foot line unless the child is unable to read that far. Record the *last* line on which the child could read three out of four symbols correctly.

11. Record the visual acuity as a fraction. The top number equals the distance the child stands from the chart. The bottom number equals the last line read satisfactorily. The average visual acuity is represented by 20/20. This means that the pupil tested reads the 20-foot line at 20 feet. *Record the visual acuity as the last line read correctly.*

12. Examples: Jane reads all the symbols on the 40-foot line; she misses two out of six on the 30-foot line and misses three out of six on the 20-foot line. Her acuity is recorded as 20/30 because the 30-foot line was the last line from which she could read four out of six symbols correctly. Jim misses two symbols on the 40-foot line so the screener moves up to the 100-foot line and then screens downward to find the last line on which he can read three out of four symbols (or four out of six) correctly. This is his acuity.

13. The recorder should observe the pupil's eyes closely during the screening for redness, squint, eye deviation, or signs of strain. Deviations from normal should be recorded.

14. If a child screens 40 or worse wearing glasses, please note the date of the last professional eye examination and doctor's name, if known.

Criteria for referrals to specialist

1. Refer the child *only* after a second screening has been made. Referrals made on the basis of one screening only too frequently result in error.

2. Rescreen those pupils who are unable to follow instructions or any pupil for whom there were questionable findings on the second screening.

3. A *second screening* should be done on all *kindergarten through third-grade* children who screened 20/40 or worse in one or both eyes.

4. A *second screening* should be done on all *fourth- through sixth-grade* children who screened 20/30 or worse in *both* eyes, or 20/40 or worse in one or both eyes.

5. *Refer* all children verified by the second screening to have 20/30 or worse in *both eyes,* or 20/40 or worse in one or both eyes, *fourth through sixth grade.*

6. *Refer* all children verified by the second screening to have 20/40 or worse in one or both eyes, *kindergarten through third grade.*

7. *Refer* all children verified by the second screening who are not under periodic eye supervision and have broken or lost their glasses, except those listed below.

8. *Do not* refer a pupil with 20/30 vision who already wears glasses if this is a recent correction. Be sure these facts are indicated on the recording sheet.

9. *Do not* refer a pupil who has had a recent eye examination and correction or a child whose eyes a doctor has indicated cannot be helped with glasses. Be sure these facts are recorded.

10. *Do not* refer a pupil who was checked without his glasses; rescreen him on a day he wears them.

Administration and scoring of the
Preschool Readiness Experimental Screening Scale (PRESS)*

Introduction. As the child is placed on the examining table and the records and equipment are organized, the following is said:
1. "Mrs. Smith, as I examine Johnny I will be asking him a few questions, so please don't talk to him for a few minutes." I smile and ask: "O.K.?"
2. "Johnny, I hear you're going to start kindergarten soon. Do you think you'll like that?"

Knowledge of colors. These questions are asked during the EENT exam.
1. "I hear your teacher will want you to know colors. Do you know any colors yet?"
2. "If she asks you to color a house, *what color should you make the grass?*"
3. *"And what color should you make the sky if there are no clouds?"*

NAME _____ BIRTHDATE _____

SCHOOL _____ DATE _____

1. a. What color is grass? _____
   b. What color is the sky if there are no clouds? _____

2. a. Repeat four numbers (one success in two tries): 4-1-7-3 or 3-8-6-4. _____
   b. Recognize four tongue blades. _____

3. a. Does Christmas come in the winter or the summer? _____
   b. Where is your heel? _____

4. Draw a square (best success in two tries). _____

5. a. Comprehension and performance. _____
   b. Personal-social maturity. _____

   TOTAL _____

Comments

PRESS General Outline and Record Form. The children were asked to reproduce a standard 1-inch square.

*From Rogers, W. B., Jr., and Rogers, R. A.: Clin. Pediatr. **11**:10, Oct. 1972; and Rogers, W. B., Jr., and Rogers, R. A.: Clin. Pediatr. **14**:253, March 1975.

Continued.

THE PRESCHOOL READINESS EXPERIMENTAL SCREENING SCALE (PRESS)

The screening scale described on the following pages is intended to provide an estimate of a 5-year-old child's readiness to enter the standard academic programs offered in most American communities. The ability to perform each of the items on this scale does not indicate specific proficiencies, but a child's inability to perform as defined in the scoring system described does give an indication of a need for specialist evaluation of the child's development and capacity before entering kindergarten or first grade. The test does not indicate intelligence or ability but simply suggests a child's general readiness to perform the usual tasks required in the school setting.

Administration and scoring of the Preschool Readiness Experimental Screening Scale (PRESS)—cont'd

Knowledge of numbers. Asked during the heart and lung exam.
1. "If the teacher tells you some numbers, could you remember them and repeat them back to her?"
2. *"I'm going to tell you some numbers. Now you remember them and say the same numbers right back to me."* (4-1-7-3 and 3-8-6-4)
3. "If the teacher asks you to count, could you do that?"
4. *"Tell me, how many tongue blades are there?"* At this point place four tongue blades on the table beside the patient.

General knowledge. As the abdomen, genitalia, and extremities are examined.
1. "I'm going to examine your tummy. You know where your tummy is, don't you?" or "Do you have a tickly tummy?"
2. *"Tell me, does Christmas come in the winter or the summer?"*
2. *"Can you show me where your heel is?"*

Drawing coordination. This is usually done at the end of the exam.
1. "If the teacher asked you to draw a square like this one (indicate the sample square), *let's see you draw one just like it right beside mine.* Take your time and make a good one."

General assessment: performance and maturity. These are best evaluated following the hearing and visual acuity tests when everything else is finished.

Scoring
COLORS. 1 point for knowing grass is green. 1 point for knowing the sky is blue. Any other answer, such as white, blue and white, or black, gets no point.

NUMBERS. 1 point for repeating the four numbers in the same sequence. If the child misses the first set of numbers, try the second set. Score 1 point for *either* set of numbers repeated back correctly. 1 point for answering the correct number of tongue blades as four. If the child only counts "one, two, three, four," this is not given a point. You may then ask the child *one time only,* "Yes, but how many are there all together?" If the child does not answer four at this time, score 0.

GENERAL KNOWLEDGE. 1 point for answering *winter.* It is important to suggest winter first. Most children will give the second of two choices if they do not know the correct answer. 1 point for knowing the heel. The child must point to the heel or the Achilles tendon, not to the malleolus.

DRAWING COORDINATION. Allow the child to draw a second square if the first one is poorly done. Encourage him to make the second more like the sample. Choosing the best square, score in the following manner:
2 points for drawing a good, readily recognizable square.

Administration and scoring of the
Preschool Readiness Experimental Screening Scale (PRESS)—cont'd

1 point for drawing a fairly recognizable square.

0 points for drawing a poor, unrecognizable square.

COMPREHENSION AND PERFORMANCE. 1 point for those who reply promptly and follow instructions well (e.g., during the hearing and visual acuity tests). 0 points for those who have to be coaxed, need frequent repetition of instructions, or need repeated clarification of what you ask.

PERSON-SOCIAL MATURITY. 1 point if the child seems reasonably mature and self-confident. 0 points for:

Excessive silliness or playing around.

Overtalkative or hyperactive.

Uncooperative, evasive, no interest.

Unduly attached to mother.

Generally immature compared with most 5-year-olds you see.

It should be evident that the PRESS is not so much a standardized test with strict rules of administration as it is a set of standardized questions that can be blended into a physical examination. One should note that it includes a few questions that are asked but not scored. These questions establish rapport and put the child at ease. They also serve as a lead-in to the test questions and serve indirectly in assessing the child's general maturity. The physician [or nurse] may intersperse or substitute other lead-in questions if he feels they would better express his method of dealing with children. It is important to ask the parent not to speak, else an oversolicitious mother may interfere by offering help and encouragement.

Rating system

1. *A score of 9 or 10 indicates high average to above average school readiness.* A child in this score range should have no difficulty doing average or above average school work.
2. *A score of 7 or 8 indicates average school readiness.* A child in this score range should have little difficulty doing average school work.
3. *A score of 6 indicates borderline school readiness.* About half of the males and about a fourth of the females with this score may have difficulty in school. It is recommended that close liaison be maintained with the teacher. If at any time the child is not functioning at class level, further study should be made at once.
4. *A score of 5 or less indicates insufficient school readiness.* Such children should be referred to a school psychologist or diagnostic center for further psychologic evaluation.

IMMUNIZATION SCHEDULES

Table 4-12. American Academy of Pediatrics recommended immunization schedule for infants, 1974*

Age	Immunizations
2 months	Diphtheria, tetanus, pertussis (DTP) Trivalent oral polio vaccine (TOPV)
4 months	DTP, TOPV
6 months	DTP, TOPV
15 months	Measles, rubella, mumps Tuberculin skin test
18 months	DTP, TOPV
4-6 years	DTP, TOPV
14-16 years	Diphtheria, tetanus (Repeat every 10 years thereafter)

*Current recommendations and information available from the American Academy of Pediatrics, P.O. Box 1034, Evanston, Ill. 60204. Also refer to Powell, K. R.: Pediatr. Nurs. **3:**7, Sept./Oct. 1977.

Table 4-13. Recommendations of the American Academy of Pediatrics for immunization of children not immunized during infancy*

Time interval	Immunizations
First visit	Diphtheria, tetanus, pertussis (DTP) Trivalent oral polio vaccine (TOPV) Tuberculin skin test
1 month later	Measles, rubella, mumps
2 months later	DTP, TOPV
4 months later	DTP, TOPV
6-12 months later	DTP, TOPV
Age 14-16 years	Tetanus, diphtheria (Repeat every 10 years thereafter)

*Report of the Committee on Infectious Disease, American Academy of Pediatrics, 1974. For current recommendations, contact the American Academy of Pediatrics, P.O. Box 1034, Evanston, Ill. 60204.

DENTAL HEALTH CARE

Prevention of dental caries is a major concern during early childhood. This is because the diet of the young child changes dramatically and often begins to include frequent snacks and because the child acquires a full first set of teeth, creating the need for beginning oral hygiene. The dangers of prolonged sucking on a bottle should be discussed with the parent if bottle feeding at bedtime or naptime continues during toddlerhood. The nutrition assessment provides information regarding the frequency and amount of carbohydrate intake. The family should be counseled in accord with this assessment and encouraged to use snacks that do not promote tooth decay, such as fresh fruit, vegetables, nuts, cheese, popcorn, milk, pretzels, and sugar-free drinks.

Table 4-14. Suggested schedule for preventive child dental health care*

Age	Developmental landmarks	Discussion and guidance	Procedures
Prenatal period		Parent education to dental needs Effect of drugs on developing dentition during pregnancy Diet and proper dental habit	Brochures and pamphlets from American Dental Association; fluoridated drinking water
Newborn	Edentulous gumpads Infantile swallowing pattern	Parent education to dental needs Effect of drugs on developing dentition during pregnancy Diet and proper dental habit Congenital anomalies Birth trauma	Thorough oral examination by obstetrician, pediatrician, etc.
Birth to 6 months	Neonatal teeth Lower deciduous incisor eruption Epstein pearls	Parent education to dental needs Effect of drugs on developing dentition during pregnancy Diet and proper dental habit Congenital anomalies Dental arch and dentitional development	Fluoridated drinking water
6 to 30 months	Correct eruption sequence and time of eruption Completion of deciduous dentition Transitional period from infantile to mature swallow Tongue, lip, finger habits Learning and sleeping habits	Effect of drugs on developing dentition during pregnancy Diet and proper dental habit Dental arch and dentitional development Traumatic injuries Oral habit patterns	Oral hygiene Oral habit control Dietary regimen check
30 months to 6 years	Complete deciduous dentition Appearance of spaces between incisor teeth	Period of use of complete deciduous dentition and developmental preparation for permanent teeth Routine periodic visits to the dentist Oral manifestations of medication and drug therapy Traumatic injuries more likely Temporomandibular joint disturbances (bruxism, clenching, rheumatoid arthritis, etc.) Dietary regimen	First visit to dentist Supervision of dental occlusion and development (arch and jaw relationships and space control) Control of abnormal pressure habits Caries control procedures Oral hygiene instruction
6 to 12 years	Mixed dentition period Eruption of eight permanent incisors and four permanent molars by 8½ years Loss of deciduous molars, eruption of premolars by 10½ to 12 years Eruption of second molars (12 year molars)	Periodic dental visits (at least twice a year) Caries, soft tissue problems Malocclusion Oral manifestations of medication and drug therapy Traumatic injuries more likely Temporomandibular joint disturbances (bruxism, clenching, rheumatoid arthritis, etc.) Dietary regimen Oral effects of endocrine activity	Supervision of dental development (arch and jaw relationships and space control) Optimal time for orthodontic consultation and guidance; possible interceptive procedures Oral hygiene instruction Caries control Soft tissue care

*Joint statement prepared by a committee of representatives from the American Academy of Pedodontics, the American Society of Dentistry for Children, the American Association of Orthodontists, and the American Academy of Pediatrics, Sept. 1966. From Standards of child health care, Evanston, Ill., 1967, American Academy of Pediatrics, p. 115.

Continued.

Table 4-14. Suggested schedule for preventive child dental health care—cont'd

Age	Developmental landmarks	Discussion and guidance	Procedures
12 to 19 years	Completion of permanent dentition Possible third molar eruption (girls first)	Periodic dental visits (at least twice a year) Caries, soft tissue problems Malocclusion Oral manifestations of medication and drug therapy Traumatic injuries more likely Temporomandibular joint disturbances (bruxism, clenching, rheumatoid arthritis, etc.) Dietary regimen Oral effects of endocrine activity	Supervision of dental development (arch and jaw relationships and space control) Optimal time for orthodontic consultation and guidance; possible interceptive procedures Oral hygiene instruction Caries control Soft tissue care Active orthodontic therapy Replacement of missing teeth Esthetic and functional considerations

DEVELOPMENT OF SECONDARY SEX CHARACTERISTICS

Table 4-15. Developmental stages of secondary sex characteristics*

Stage	Male genital development	Male and female pubic hair development	Female breast development	Other changes
1	Prepuberty	Prepuberty; hair over the pubic area similar to that on the abdomen	Prepuberty; increased pigmentation of the papillae only	
2	Initial enlargement of the scrotum and testes; reddening and texture changes of the scrotum	Sparse growth of long, straight, downy hair at the base of the penis or along the labia	Enlargement of areolar diameter; small area of elevation around the papillae	Usual time of peak height velocity for girls
3	Initial enlargement of the penis; further growth of testes and scrotum	Hair becomes darker, more coarse, and curly; spreads sparsely over the entire pubic area	Further elevation and enlargement of breasts and areolas, with no separation of the contours	Usual point of onset of menstruation Facial hair begins to grow and voice deepens for boys
4	Further enlargement of the penis, testes, and scrotum; growth in breadth and development of the glans	Further spread of hair distribution not extending to the thighs	Areolas and papillae project from the breast to form a secondary mound	Usual time of peak height velocity for boys Auxiliary hair begins to grow
5	Adult in size and contour	Adult in amount and type	Adult, with projection of the papillae only; recession of the areolas into the general breast contour	

*As defined by Tanner, J. M.: Growth at adolescence, ed. 2, Oxford, 1962, Blackwell Scientific Publications, Ltd.

ENVIRONMENTAL STANDARDS

Environmental standards for pollutants are given in Table 4-16. Standards* for the fluoridation of water are:

0.6 ppm—not sufficient.

0.7 to 1.5 ppm—optimal range.

Over 1.5—fluoride content should be reduced.

---

*These are not federal standards. They were proposed by Dr. John W. Knutson, former Chief Dental Officer, Public Health Service.

Table 4-16. Federal environmental standards*

Pollutant	Period	Federal air standards (ambient)	
		Primary	Secondary
Particulate	Annual (geometric mean)	75µg/cu meter	60µg/cu meter
	24 hours	260µg/cu meter†	·150µg/cu meter†
Sulfur oxides	Annual (arithmetic mean)	0.03 ppm	0.02 ppm
	24 hours	0.14 ppm†	0.10 ppm†‡
	3 hours	—	0.50 ppm†
Carbon monoxide	8 hours (running average)	9 ppm†	Same as primary
	1 hour	35 ppm†	Same as primary
Oxidants	1 hour	0.08 ppm†	Same as primary
Hydrocarbons	3 hours	0.24 ppm†§	Same as primary
Nitrogen oxides	Annual (arithmetic mean)	0.05 ppm	Same as primary

*As a guide to be used in assessing implementation plans for achieving the annual maximum 24-hour standard.
†Value not to be exceeded more than once per year.
‡As a guide to be used in assessing implementation plans for achieving the annual arithmetic mean standard.
§As a guide in devising implementation plans for achieving oxidant standards.

CHAPTER 5

Criteria for hospitalization and home care

CRITERIA FOR HOSPITALIZATION*

Four major risks have been identified with hospitalization of children:

1. Emotional and separation problems, particularly for children under 4 years of age, can be transient or permanent, but they are significant for the child and the family.
2. The parents' confidence in their own ability to care for the child themselves may be undermined.
3. Exposure to infection is increased in the hospital setting.
4. The family and society sustain a significant economic cost, which, for the family, may constitute a lasting stress.

---

*Material from this section prepared with reference to the following: Hardgrove, C. B., and Dawson, R. B.: Parents and children in the hospital; the family's role in pediatrics, Boston, 1972, Little, Brown & Co.,; Vernon, D. T., and others: The psychological responses of children to hospitalization and illness; a review of the literature, Springfield, Ill., 1965, Charles C Thomas, Publisher; Schmitt, B. D., Duncan, B. R., and Riley, C. M.: Ambulatory pediatrics. In Kempe, C. H., Silver, H. K., and O'Brien, D., editors: Current pediatric diagnosis and treatment, ed. 2, Los Altos, Calif., 1972, Lange Medical Publications, p. 123; Gardner, P., and Carles, D. G.: Infections acquired in a pediatric hospital, J. Pediatr. **81:**1205-1210, Dec. 1972; and Freiberg, K. H.: How parents react when their child is hospitalized, Am. J. Nurs. **72:**1270-1272, July 1972.

When hospitalization is clearly required, these risks must be considered in terms of compensation during the hospitalization itself. When indications for hospitalization are less clear, they are weighed against the evidence for hospitalization and the real ability of the family to care for the child at home. Thus it is helpful to consider carefully the criteria on which the decision to hospitalize a child is based. Although this decision is most often a medical one, all health care workers should be familiar with the criteria so that they may contribute to the gathering of relevant information on which to base a decision, facilitate optimal care, and help avoid delays in taking appropriate steps.

There are three classes of criteria for hospitalization of a child: (1) major emergencies, (2) potentially life-threatening or crippling illness, and (3) specific psychosocial indications.

Major emergencies

Major emergencies are clear life-threatening circumstances such as shock, severe dehydration, coma; signs of major acute illness such as meningitis, respiratory distress, epiglottitis, renal failure, severe poisonings; life-threating accidents such as extensive burns or head injury; and surgical emergencies. The single criterion that applies universally is that the condition is life-threatening.

Potentially life-threatening or crippling illness

Criteria for these illnesses are less easily formulated, since the extent of a problem may be difficult or impossible to delineate. Specific criteria for use by all members of the health care team should be developed to fit the preferences of the team members and the particular situation. The following guidelines are offered to assist in the development of more specific criteria for conditions commonly encountered in a given setting.

Age and stage of development

In infants there is a greater risk that physiologic imbalance will occur quickly and threaten life. Such conditions as diarrhea, cellulitis, bleeding, respiratory tract infection (for example, pneumonia), renal malfunction, or any suspicious condition that is not possible to fully describe without the specific resources of the hospital indicate the need for hospitalization. After the separation anxiety phenomenon has occured, the infant has gained enough of an advantage in maintaining physiologic imbalance that hospitalization might be delayed if the family can adequately care for the child at home and can understand all aspects of treatment needed. It is at this point that the child's emotional response to hospitalization becomes a serious risk, and hospitalization should be avoided if at all possible.

Illness factors

Illness that is not a major emergency but that may potentially become life-threatening is difficult to separate from illness that will not progress into a more serious condition. The guidelines that might be developed for specific conditions may be somewhat arbitrary, and experience is needed in a particular setting to judge the adequacy of specified guidelines. The following are offered as examples.

Burns. The child who suffers (1) burns involving more than 10% to 15% of total body area (Fig. 5-1), (2) burns involving the perineal area or the hands, or (3) electrical burns should be hospitalized.

Respiratory tract infections. Any child who has an infection involving the respiratory tract that causes respiratory distress or potentially involves respiratory distress (such as diphtheria, pertussis) or who has complications such as hemoptysis, mastoiditis, anemia, or history of previous severe respiratory distress requires hospitalization.

Head injury. Children who suffer head injury without apparent skull fracture and who are unconscious longer than 1 minute, have persistent neurologic signs such as disorientation, irritability, decreased consciousness level, or headaches, or exhibit bleeding from any orifice of the head should be hospitalized.

Febrile seizures. If the seizure lasts for longer than 5 to 10 minutes or if neurologic signs persist and consciousness level is decreased, the child should be hospitalized for the remainder of the febrile illness and for possible diagnostic investigation.

In addition, any child whose illness is managed at home and does not begin to respond within 2 days of the onset of treatment should be considered for hospitalization.

Diagnostic factors

This criterion is particularly susceptible to misuse because there are many instances when a child's signs and symptoms are extremely elusive and the child is subjected to hospitalization in a desire to fully delineate the nature of the problem. This can arise from the preference of either the physician or the family. Although there are many instances that fully warrant such an approach, every effort should be made to avoid hospitalizing simply for diagnostic purposes. Diagnoses can often be accomplished through office and clinic facilities, but insurance policies currently held by many families do not provide for such diagnostic services. Unless the family is suffering from undue financial strain, the child should not be hospitalized because of insurance considerations alone.

Suspected illnesses that definitely warrant full diagnostic exploration within the hospital setting tend to meet specific guidelines. First, there are those that are amenable to specific treatment if discovered early and adequate treatment is begun promptly. Examples include such illnesses as pyelonephritis, thrombophle-

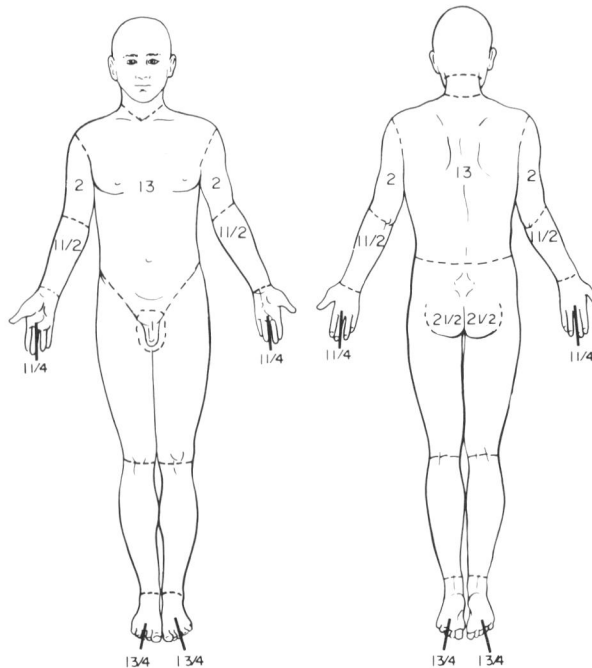

Relative percentages of areas affected by growth

AREA	Inf	1-4	5-9	10-14	15	Adult	Part	Full	Total	Donor areas
HEAD	19	17	13	11	9	7				
NECK	2	2	2	2	2	2				
ANT TRUNK	13	13	13	13	13	13				
POST TRUNK	13	13	13	13	13	13				
R BUTTOCK	$2\frac{1}{2}$	$2\frac{1}{2}$	$2\frac{1}{2}$	$2\frac{1}{2}$	$2\frac{1}{2}$	$2\frac{1}{2}$				
L BUTTOCK	$2\frac{1}{2}$	$2\frac{1}{2}$	$2\frac{1}{2}$	$2\frac{1}{2}$	$2\frac{1}{2}$	$2\frac{1}{2}$				
GENITALIA	1	1	1	1	1	1				
R U ARM	4	4	4	4	4	4				
L U ARM	4	4	4	4	4	4				
R L ARM	3	3	3	3	3	3				
L L ARM	3	3	3	3	3	3				
R HAND	$2\frac{1}{2}$	$2\frac{1}{2}$	$2\frac{1}{2}$	$2\frac{1}{2}$	$2\frac{1}{2}$	$2\frac{1}{2}$				
L HAND	$2\frac{1}{2}$	$2\frac{1}{2}$	$2\frac{1}{2}$	$2\frac{1}{2}$	$2\frac{1}{2}$	$2\frac{1}{2}$				
R THIGH	$5\frac{1}{2}$	$6\frac{1}{2}$	8	$8\frac{1}{2}$	9	$9\frac{1}{2}$				
L THIGH	$5\frac{1}{2}$	$6\frac{1}{2}$	8	$8\frac{1}{2}$	9	$9\frac{1}{2}$				
R LEG	5	5	$5\frac{1}{2}$	6	$6\frac{1}{2}$	7				
L LEG	5	5	$5\frac{1}{2}$	6	$6\frac{1}{2}$	7				
R FOOT	$3\frac{1}{2}$	$3\frac{1}{2}$	$3\frac{1}{2}$	$3\frac{1}{2}$	$3\frac{1}{2}$	$3\frac{1}{2}$				
L FOOT	$3\frac{1}{2}$	$3\frac{1}{2}$	$3\frac{1}{2}$	$3\frac{1}{2}$	$3\frac{1}{2}$	$3\frac{1}{2}$				
						TOTAL				

Fig. 5-1. Burn estimate diagram. (From Chinn, P. L.: Child health maintenance; concepts in family-centered care, ed. 2, St. Louis, 1979, The C. V. Mosby Co. After Jacoby, F. G.: Nursing care of the patient with burns, ed. 2, St. Louis, 1976, The C. V. Mosby Co.)

bitis, acute rheumatic fever, rheumatoid arthritis, osteomyelitis, lead poisoning, and failure to thrive. Second, a condition may require the specific setting of the hospital in order to conduct the diagnostic tests. Hospitalization is often justified because special preparation is necessary for the tests, specific observation must be made of the recovery after the tests, or the tests require a surgical procedure.

Specific psychosocial indications

These indications arise primarily from a community's limitations in offering health care services during specific crisis situations. As resources of the community expand to help families with specific health care problems, the need for hospitalization decreases. The following guidelines should be used in developing criteria for specific conditions, and the community resources should be considered as alternatives to hospitalization as they are available.

Parent factors

When a child has a health problem of any proportion and the criteria for home care cannot be met (see following section), hospitalization is required to provide adequate care for the time being. Such problems include suspected or confirmed child abuse or neglect, severe economic deprivation, parental physical exhaustion, emotional incapacitation of one or both parents, or intellectually limited parents.

Child factors

When a child has a problem that is not manageable at home or that arises from the home situation, hospitalization may be indicated. Emotional incapacitation of the child, emotional disturbance or crisis such as a suicide attempt, or socially dangerous or unduly disruptive behavior may be an indication for hospitalization until the crisis passes, therapy has been instituted, or some alternative plan to returning to the home can be implemented.

Illness factors

There are three conditions that commonly lead to hospitalization even though none of the other criteria are met.

Initial diagnosis of an illness requiring a complex treatment regimen. Even though the treatment is conducted at home throughout the remainder of the illness or the child's life, initial teaching and supervision may require the full concentration of the health care team in the hospital setting. For example, juvenile-onset diabetes mellitus requires a careful, deliberate, organized child- and family-centered program of teaching and support in learning to administer insulin and to balance all other aspects of life. Some communities have begun to develop centers for intensive provision of such teaching and guidance programs as alternatives to hospitalization. Such a program offers the advantages of more closely resembling the home setting,

providing daily activities that simulate those experienced in everyday living, and making available a team of specialized health care workers who center on the specific health problem of the individual.

Initial diagnosis of a fatal illness. Hospitalization in such a case may be necessary for psychosocial reasons alone. The family and the child may require the extra support and assistance found within the hospital as they work through the initial impact of the diagnosis.

Terminal care of the dying child. Terminal care may be required if the family needs the support of the hospital health care team during this phase of illness or if they prefer that the child not die at home. Although it is usually possible to care for the dying child in the home, the stress and burden of physical care added to the burden of the emotional situation is more than some families can bear.

CRITERIA FOR HOME CARE

When criteria for hospitalization are not clearly met, the following criteria for home care should be fully explored by the health care worker and the family.

Personal resources of the parents

In order for a child to remain in the home for care during an illness, there must be an adult present in the home who can give the physical and emotional care required. In addition, there should be resources for obtaining relief from the physical burden of care so that each adult involved in care has the opportunity for sleep and rest and for some diversion from the illness of the child, particularly if the illness is prolonged. Adults caring for the child should have the capacity to understand the nature of the illness and the care and treatment regimen needed, and they should demonstrate the needed skill in admisistering required treatment.

Physical environment of the home

The home should be reasonably conducive to the physical requirements of the child. There should be facilities for washing, elimination, food preparation, and reasonable diversion and entertainment for the child. The home should also be reasonably convenient for those who must care for the child and operate the household. There should be an indication that physical safety from injury or infection can be maintained throughout the illness or treatment period. For example, if the child requires humidification added to the room with an electrical device, the electrical facilities of the home should appear safe and there should be reasonable assurance that the family is able to consider the safety requirements of using such a device.

Social environment of the home

The presence of siblings or other relatives in the home may constitute an advantage or a disadvantage in home care of an ill child. If there are several young siblings who require a great deal of attention and care, the mother may not be able to care for a sick child. On the other hand, if siblings can participate in certain aspects of the child's care, if they can understand the child's needs for rest, treatment, or extra attention, and if there is no threat to the health of the siblings, they may provide a desirable contribution to the total care of the child. Adult relatives in the home may provide needed help in the physical and emotional burdens of caring for the ill child, or they may present a barrier to providing adequate care.

The interpersonal atmosphere should be reasonably harmonious and congruent with the goals of healthy living. A family that is ordinarily able to maintain its basic form and to cope with problems of everyday living or occasional extraordinary stress is ideally suited to caring for the ill child at home. Families that experience periodic stages of disorganization, have borderline ability to cope with extraordinary stress, or seem to create interpersonal stress among the members may respond favorably to the stress of a child's illness and gather together all of their positive resources to center on the needs of the child. The crisis may serve as a unifying force bringing the family together; or it may provide the stimulus that breaks the ties that have tenuously held the family unit together. When factors such as these are difficult to ascertain, the judgment must be made with the family regarding a possible trial in caring for the child at home or turning to hospitalization from the outset. It must be acknowledged that hospitalization of the child may produce stress of a different kind that will affect the family's stability with an impact equal to home care; the family must decide which kind of stress they can most effectively cope with.

Supportive community resources

If the child's home meets the above requirements and any special health care needs can be met through resources in the community, home care is possible and desirable. Special nursing services, nutrition teaching and consultation, and various forms of therapy and treatment may be available either through an outpatient clinic or in the home.

CHAPTER 6

Management of common illness in childhood

The following outline is offered as a suggested guideline for the management of several common illnesses in childhood by qualified health care workers. The problems that are identified are considered appropriate nursing problems for a nurse with advanced preparation in child care. A nursing diagnosis is defined as a problem that is subject to intervention within the realm of nursing practice. Likewise, a medical diagnosis is that which requires medical intervention. The diagnostic criteria and protocols for management may be altered to suit the preferences of various health care teams. Once specific guidelines for diagnostic criteria and protocols for management have been ascertained, it is expected that all qualified health care workers will make decisions and implement care based on these guidelines, documenting their decisions and actions on behalf of each child. Consultation with another health care worker or specialist with advanced preparation may be indicated for any child whose signs and symptoms do not fully warrant a given problem outlined in the guide. For a complete discussion of nursing management of illness in childhood, see *Child Health Maintenance: Concepts in Family-Centered Care,** Chapters 11, 13, 15, and 18.

---

*Chinn, P. L.: St. Louis, 1979, The C. V. Mosby Co.

Table 6-1. Common illnesses in childhood

Problem	Diagnostic criteria	Protocol for management

Fever	Body temperature measured to be above 101° F accompanied by signs of systemic illness and/or persisting for several hours.
	NURSING DIAGNOSIS
	1. Fever of relatively brief duration before the diagnostic encounter (usually less than 24-hour history) and onset and continuance are accompanied by symptoms of minor childhood illness, which is also identified and documented.
	2. Fever has not persisted beyond 104° F and responds readily to treatment. In addition, fever does not persist beyond the point that related symptoms of illness begin to subside.
	3. No history of febrile convulsions.
	MEDICAL DIAGNOSIS
	When the above criteria are not documented, fever is clearly a medical problem and requires medical diagnosis. The primary problem will usually become one of diagnosis of the underlying cause of the fever, which is beyond the scope of this outline.
		1. Appropriate treatment for related illness.
		2. Symptomatic relief of fever.
		  a. Environmental measures to increase body heat loss, such as sponge bathing, tepid water bathing, dressing in light clothing, greater fluid intake.
		  b. Drugs for control of fever:
		    Aspirin; dosage calculated as follows:
		      Weight: 65 mg (1 gr)/kg/24 hours in 4-6 doses.
		      Surface area: 1.5 g/sq meter/24 hours in 4-6 doses.
		    Acetaminophen; dosage calculated as follows:
		      Age:
		        Under 1 year—60 mg.
		        1-3 years—60-120 mg.
		        3-6 years—120 mg.
		        Over 6 years—240 mg.
		        (Single doses repeated every 4-6 hours.)
		      Surface area: 0.7 g/sq meter/24 hours in 4-6 doses.
		  NOTE: These drugs should be used with caution in all children under 2 years of age; doses continuing beyond 24 hours should be administered by a physician.
		3. Monitor body hydration.
		  a. Obtain accurate body weight when the problem is identified.
		  b. Document state of tissue turgor.
		  c. Encourage fluid intake.

Gastrointestinal disturbances		

Colic	Infant cries vigorously as if in pain, usually after feeding or in the evening; cannot be comforted.
	1. Rule out minor constipation, anal fissure, pain with bowel movement.
		1. Active listening with insightful judgment and counseling regarding parent's perception of problem. Suggest several possible approaches depending on situation:
		  a. Keep infant warm, particularly extremities.
		  b. Take infant for a walk or ride.
		  c. Alter mother's diet if infant is breast fed.
		  d. Use mild phenobarbital preparation as last resort if infant does not respond to other measures.

	2. Rule out milk allergy.	2. Use trial formula of soy preparation for 1-2 weeks. If infant responds, continue until 3 months of age, then try milk formula once again to determine tolerance.

Table 6-1. Common illnesses in childhood—cont'd

Problem	Diagnostic criteria	Protocol for management

Gastrointestinal disturbances—cont'd

"Flu" (communicable variety with vomiting and diarrhea)

1. Subjective presence of any of the following:
   a. Abdominal cramping.
   b. Vomiting, diarrhea.
   c. Systemic symptoms such as fever, joint aches, muscle pain.
2. Objective evidence of each of the following:
   a. Fever.
   b. Community epidemiology.
   c. State of hydration; dehydration representing loss of more than 6% of body weight since onset of illness requires medical management.

NOTE: Attention must be given to possible serious illness (such as rheumatic fever, rheumatoid arthritis, ulcerative colitis, appendicitis, and so on) that may mimic the common flu, particularly in the absence of community epidemiology or when the symptoms persist or recur frequently.

1. Treat vomiting and diarrhea as follows:
   a. Discontinue all usual diet.
      Infant: prescribe Lytren or other commercial electrolyte fluid preparation for 24-48 hours. A homemade preparation may be used if parent is able to reliably prepare the following:
         1 quart of boiled water
         ½ teaspoon of salt (do not exceed)
         3 tablespoons sugar
      Child: cola, ginger ale, root beer, Jell-O water, or other clear liquids as tolerated; soda crackers as tolerated.
      All infants and children: offer small amounts of fluid (15-30 ml) frequently (every 15-20 minutes).
   b. Continue to give only clear liquids for 24-48 hours. If symptoms have not disappeared, notify nurse or physician. If symptoms have disappeared, slowly begin resuming diet, leaving milk as last food to be reintroduced. Infants on formula only may be offered boiled skim milk for 24 additional hours.
2. Monitor body hydration.
   a. Obtain accurate body weight when the problem is identified.
   b. Document state of tissue turgor and other signs of hydration (fontanel, irritability, and so on).
   c. Assure adequate fluid intake for maintenance.
3. Treat fever as above.
4. Comfort measures as needed.

Upper respiratory tract disturbances

Otitis media, uncomplicated

Definitive diagnosis requires culture of the middle ear cavity fluid. Probably diagnosis may rest on visualization of the tympanic membrane in which the following features are noted:
a. Absence of bony landmarks.
b. Absence of the light reflex.
c. Bulging or redness of the membrane.
d. Serous drainage.

1. Preferences for treatment vary among practitioners. Health care teams may select detailed guides for the use of any of the following measures:
   a. Antibiotics per MP.*
   b. Saline nose drops for symptomatic relief.
   c. Decongestant per MP.*
2. Symptomatic treatment of fever may be indicated.
3. Physician collaboration and/or management indicated when symptoms recur within a 3-month period.

*Management protocol developed by the local health care team.

Continued.

Table 6-1. Common illnesses in childhood—cont'd

Problem	Diagnostic criteria	Protocol for management
Upper respiratory tract disturbances—cont'd		

Common cold, also known as coldlike syndrome, URI, coryza, rhinitis, rhinopharyngitis, acute catarrhal tonsillo-pharyngitis	1. Objective presence of a combination of any of the following symptoms:
	  a. Nasal congestion.
	  b. Sore or "scratchy" throat.
	  c. Cough.
	  d. Sneezing.
	  e. Minimal degree of fever.
	2. Documented absence of definitive signs of infection of related structures:
	  a. Ears: tympanic membranes appear normal.
	  b. Lungs: breath sounds are normal; no congestion; breathing is not distressed.
	  c. Throat: no evidence of purulent drainage or excoriative lesions; swallowing not impaired.
	  d. Mouth: no signs of Koplik's spots on the buccal membranes (indicative of measles).
	  e. Nervous system: absence of signs of meningeal irritation.
	3. Consider possibility of:
	  a. Allergies with frequent attacks (obtain eosinophil count, try antihistamine drugs).
	  b. Foreign body in nose.
	  c. Strep infection in infant under 6 months.
	  d. Whooping cough (obtain culture).
	  e. Measles in preeruptive stage for non-immunized child.
		1. Determine parent's care to present, especially medications. Prescribe rest, force fluids, and aspirin to relieve discomfort.
		2. Other measures that may be used, particularly when prevention of lower infection is desirable, include:
		  a. Mist or steam vapor.
		  b. Postural drainage.
		  c. Antihistamines per MP.
		  d. Cough syrup per MP.
		  e. Decongestant per MP.

Acute tonsillopharyngitis With exudate ("strep throat")	1. Culture evidence of group A beta hemolytic streptococcal infection. 2. Purulent exudative tonsils. 3. Enlarged, tender nodes. 4. Fever. 5. Sudden onset of symptoms.	Antibiotic treatment per MP. Symptomatic treatment as for cold. NOTE: Prevention of rheumatic fever and other complications demands that the child receive an adequate dose of penicillin for 10 days or a long-acting bicillin or other suitable chemotherapy. A positive culture should be followed by cultures of siblings and close friends.
With membrane (possible diphtheria)	Similar to strep but membrane rather than exudate is present.	Referral for medical diagnosis and care.
With vesicles or ulcers (possible herpes simplex)	Similar to strep but with ulcers and vesicles present rather than exudate.	1. Possible smallpox vaccine. 2. Symptomatic relief of subjective symptoms. 3. Throat culture to rule out strep infection.

Table 6-1. Common illnesses in childhood—cont'd

Problem	Diagnostic criteria	Protocol for management
Lower respiratory tract disturbances		
Acute laryngitis Croup Bronchiolitis Asthma Pneumonia Whooping cough	Physician diagnosis required, and institution of medical care is mandatory. Signs that may be detected by the nurse include: a. Rales and rhonchi in chest; locate and describe. b. Pleuritic friction rub. c. Productive cough. d. Retractions. e. Expiratory grunt. f. Air hunger and oxygen deprivation.	1. Symptomatic nursing care is indicated as an adjunct to medical care. 2. Emergency MP or telephone orders are possible when the nurse is able to give thorough description of all objective symptoms, but medical consultation is required as soon as possible.
Skin problems		
Diaper rashes Thrush	1. Characteristic white spots in mouth may be detected before diaper rash appears. 2. Diaper rash has characteristic bright red, "raw meat" appearance with excoriation of skin.	Prescribe nystatin (Mycostatin) drops per MP.
Minor diaper rash	Maculopapular rash, which may or may not be confluent; ranges in color from mild pink to bright red. Some discomfort may be present.	1. Determine parent's treatment and laundering practices to date. Instruct parent regarding frequency of changes, cleansing, laundering of diapers. 2. Advise immediate rinsing of diapers and water soaking until washing without sitting over 24 hours. Use mild soap (no detergent). Reintroduce usual laundry compounds only after rash has resolved, one agent at a time. 3. Leave diaper area exposed to air as much as possible until rash resolves. Discontinue use of plastic pants; use only when necessary if rash persists intermittently. 4. Advise use of A & D ointment or, for severe, persistently repeated attacks, a preparation containing zinc oxide and/or cod liver oil.
"Cradle cap"	Flaking white material adhering to scalp.	Instruct parent in daily vigorous brushing of scalp, preferably during shampooing. Ask for return demonstration if possible. Fontanel area is a common site of initial cradle cap because of parent's fear of damaging the spot. Demonstrate and reassure regarding the use of brisk shampooing and brushing. A small toothbrush enhances effective scalp stimulation.
Dandruff	Same as cradle cap; occurs in older child or teenager.	Initial use of dandruff treatment shampoo daily or every other day until itching and flaking disappear. Thereafter, use of regular shampoo at least once a week and 2-3 times a week after puberty or if skin is unusually oily.

Continued.

Table 6-1. Common illnesses in childhood—cont'd

Problem	Diagnostic criteria	Protocol for management
Skin problems—cont'd		
Minor cuts	Any cut that does not extend beyond the dermis or subcutaneous tissue in depth or is less than 1 cm in length. EXCEPTIONS: cuts that occur in an esthetically sensitive area, such as the face.	1. Administer tetanus immunization when appropriate. 2. Cleanse the wound thoroughly. 3. If stitches are required, obtain treatment. 4. For borderline cuts or those located in an inconspicuous area, butterfly closure may suffice, leaving the wound open to air as much as possible. 5. Minor cuts should be left open to air if at all possible, with instructions to keep the area clean. Signs of infection should be taught to the child and caretaker. IN THE EVENT OF INFECTION: soak the infected area in warm water or warm moist packs 3-4 times daily. Epsom salts may be used if edema around the wound has occurred. If streaking, marked induration, or inflammation occurs, obtain physican evaluation.
Minor burns (see p. 87)	1. Less than 10% body surface involvement is often a minor burn. Severity of a burn may not be readily observable. Exceptions occur when the severity of the burn is great or when the face, perineum, or hands are involved. 2. Burns involving an extensive area or entire limb are potentially major injuries despite the initial impressions of degree of burn.	1. Emergency treatment of all burns is to expose the burned area to cold water. Burns involving an entire limb or major part of the body require immediate medical attention. 2. All persons caring for children should receive information regarding emergency care of burns and burn prevention.
Insect bites	Isolated macules or papules should be considered suspect insect bites, particularly in the presence of localized itching and stinging. Recent activities and places visited may also give a clue as to whether the condition is a bite.	1. Local relief of discomfort with alcohol, baking soda, or calamine lotion. 2. Bee, wasp, or tick bites and stings: remove the head or the stinger with tweezers. A volatile solution applied to the body of a tick facilitates removal of the head intact. 3. Systemic reactions must be halted immediately using epinephrine and/or antihistamines per MP. 4. Group-specific antivenom is available for certain spiders and scorpions.
Impetigo	1. Discrete, isolated lesions are present and tend to occur on exposed surfaces of the body, particularly those areas subject to scratches and minor cuts. 2. Early lesions are vesicular, progressing to pustular and then to a crusting stage. 3. When the crust is removed, a red, inflamed corium is exposed. 4. Systemic symptoms of illness are not present. 5. Culture evidence of streptococcal or staphylococcal infection.	1. Systemic antibiotic treatment per MP. 2. Removal of scabs by soaking and gentle washing, followed by application of local antibiotic preparation. 3. Instruction for child and family regarding skin care and hygiene or possible play areas where child may encounter unduly contaminated conditions such as animal wastes, and so on.

Table 6-1. Common illnesses in childhood—cont'd

Problem	Diagnostic criteria	Protocol for management
Skin problems—cont'd		
Acne	1. Young person has reached puberty or beyond. 2. Maculopapular lesions progress to vesicles or pustules containing either clear or dark fluid. Most often appear on face and neck; also appear on extremities and trunk.	1. Immaculate cleansing and washing 3 or 4 times daily with mild soap and water. 2. Removal of pustules and papules may be performed with a comedo remover; this procedure should not be performed by the adolescent, because scarring may result from improper removal. 3. Skin abrasives, ultraviolet light, and topical medications may be used per MP. 4. Counseling and guidance related to cosmetic selection and use. 5. Dietary trials and challenges may be attempted if young person is able to do so. 6. In severe instances, dermatologic assistance is required, and professional counseling may be indicated.
Systemic problems manifested in the skin		
Chickenpox	1. Prodomal period: may not occur in young children; older children may have 1-2 days of fever, headache, malaise, anorexia. 2. Rash: rapid evolution of initial macules to papules to vesicles and finally to crusts. Greatest density on the trunk. 3. Accompanying signs of illness are usually absent or minor.	1. Comfort measures for itching. 2. Symptomatic relief of accompanying signs and symptoms, such as fever, anorexia. 3. Isolation from susceptible children and adults from onset until all vesicles have reached the crust stage.
Enteroviral infection	1. Prodromal period: none or moderate fever and irritability for 3 or 4 days. 2. Rash: maculopapular, discrete, not itchy, evenly distributed over entire body. 3. Most common in fall and summer months. Minor signs of illness, if any, occur.	Symptomatic treatment for signs and symptoms, if any.
Erythema infectiosum	1. Prodromal period: none. 2. Rash: red, flushed cheeks (slapped face appearance) followed by a maculopapular rash in a lacelike pattern that may be precipitated for several days by various irritants, including sunlight. 3. Usually there are no accompanying signs of illness.	Symptomatic treatment as indicated.
Exanthema subitum (roseola)	1. Prodromal period: 3 or 4 days with high fever (104° F or higher) and irritability. 2. Rash: rose-red maculopapular rash that usually appears first on the chest and trunk and then spreads over the face and extremities, lasting for several hours to 2 days. 3. When the rash appears, the prodromal fever suddenly subsides and the child feels better.	Symptomatic treatment for fever during prodromal period; children who are under 2 years of age (age of greatest occurrence) who may have been exposed may be isolated during an attack of high fever in the event that roseola is in progress.

Continued.

Table 6-1. Common illnesses in childhood—cont'd

Problem	Diagnostic criteria	Protocol for management
Systemic problems manifested in the skin—cont'd		
Measles (rubeola)	1. Prodromal period: 3-4 days of fever, conjunctivitis, coryza, cough; Koplik's spots in the buccal membranes may be noted. 2. Rash: reddish brown maculopapular rash that first appears on the face and neck, progressing to the trunk and extremities.	1. Isolation during the prodromal period and 1 week after the appearance of the rash. 2. Symptomatic treatment of signs of illness, including fever, photophobia, anorexia, and so on.
Scarlet fever	1. Prodromal period: fever, sore throat, and vomiting within 12 hours before the onset of the rash. 2. Rash: erythematous punctiform lesions that blanch on pressure. Appears first on the flexural surfaces of the arms, legs, and groin, and quickly becomes generalized, involving the hands and feet. 3. Tongue appears strawberry red; exudative or membranous tonsillitis often present. Group A beta hemolytic streptococci may be cultured from the throat. 4. By fifth day the rash begins to fade, with brownish staining and desquamation. NOTE: Children who have been immunized may exhibit a mild, unusual form of the illness that mimics Rocky Mountain spotted fever.	1. Antibiotic treatment is essential. 2. Symptomatic relief for discomfort and signs of illness. 3. Obtain cultures from all persons in intimate contact. 4. Signs of meningeal irritation or other complications require immediate medical attention.
Rocky Mountain spotted fever	1. Prodromal period: 3-4 days of fever, chills, headache, joint pain, malaise, and anorexia. 2. Rash: maculopapular and petechial, with a centrifugal distribution. Palms of hands and soles of feet may be involved. 3. Recent history of tick bite. 4. Nervous system and cardiovascular system involvement occurs in about 20% of all persons infected. 5. Definitive diagnosis available through a specific Rocky Mountain spotted fever complement fixation test.	1. Antibiotic treatment required to prevent major complications and fatality. 2. Symptomatic relief of signs of illness; medical diagnosis and management required.
Rubella	1. Prodromal period: none, or mild lymphadenopathy, low grade fever, malaise for 1-4 days. 2. Rash: pink maculopapular rash beginning on the face and neck and progressing downward to the trunk and extremities within 48 hours. 3. No accompanying signs of illness in young children; older children or adults have fever, lymphadenopathy, and joint pain. 4. Positive throat culture of the rubella virus may be obtained.	1. Symptomatic treatment. 2. Isolation, particularly from all nonimmunized, susceptible pregnant women in the first trimester.

Table 6-1. Common illnesses in childhood—cont'd

Problem	Diagnostic criteria	Protocol for management
Accidental injury		

Head injury	1. History of injury, which probably affected the head; objective evidence of injury to the scalp, skull, and/or nervous system is usually present.
	2. Documentation of nature of injury includes:
	   a. Determination of nature of the accident and child's immediate response, including length of unconsciousness, if any.
	   b. Nature of behavior and alertness following initial reaction.
	   c. Pulse, respiration, and blood pressure noted and followed for at least an hour.
	   d. Presence of reflexes and neurologic signs appropriate for age, including the nature of each response.
	   e. Eyegrounds, nasal passages, and ear canal and tympanic membranes inspected for possible signs of intracranial pressure or bleeding.
		1. Hospitalization required if unconsciousness lasts more than 3 minutes immediately following the injury.
		2. Discontinue use of all drugs that might mask symptoms of intracranial injury (discontinuing long-term medication requires medical judgment).
		3. Aspirin in appropriate doses may be used for older children who suffer headache after a minor injury.

Accidental poisoning	History of ingestion, or physical signs suggesting poison ingestion.	1. Contact local poison control center for advance information and preparation if child is to be transported. 2. Administer 15 ml syrup of ipecac to induce vomiting; repeat dose in 20 minutes if vomiting does not occur. 3. In case of ingestion of caustic substance, administer activated charcoal and transport to emergency setting for removal. 4. Obtain sample of material ingested and/or vomitus for analysis. 5. Transport to emergency setting or observe at home.
Venereal disease		
Syphilis, congenital or acquired	1. Definitive diagnosis depends on identification of the spirochete by microscopic dark-field examination of exudate from lesions or by special diagnostic tests of blood or spinal fluid. 2. Suggestive diagnostic clues include: a. Presence of lesion or chancre at the sight of entry of the organism on the skin (acquired instances only). Appearance of lesion is variable but often resembles ulcerated area surrounded by a firm, raised border. Ulcerated portion and its exudate are highly infectious.	1. Antibiotic treatment per MP. 2. Obtain history of intimate contact during periods of contagion; refer to public health agency for appropriate follow-through. 3. Counseling and guidance as indicated for emotional and social problems.

Continued.

Table 6-1. Common illnesses in childhood—cont'd

Problem	Diagnostic criteria	Protocol for management
	b. Generalized or localized lesions on the skin indicate advanced stage of infection. Rash often involves palms of the hands and soles of the feet and may resemble chickenpox, measles, or scarlet fever. Accompanying signs of illness include fever, swollen or painful lymph nodes, headache, bone and joint pain, sore throat, hair loss, eye inflammation, jaundice, albumin in the urine, or signs of meningeal irritation. These signs may appear in the young child who has congenital syphilis; in addition, the young child may have symptoms that resemble a common cold, and development, including bone and tooth development, may be unusual. c. History of sexual contact with an infected partner.	

Gonorrhea	1. Definitive diagnosis depends on laboratory culture of *Neisseria gonorrhoeae* from discharges of the male urethra or the female cervical os.
	2. Suggestive diagnostic clues include:
	  a. Men: sudden onset of thin, watery white discharge from the urethra accompanied by burning during urination. The discharge becomes thick and yellow within a day of onset.
	  b. Women: seldom exhibit bothersome symptoms of early stages of infection; may have mild cervicitis and vaginal discharge. Knowledge of infection in a sexual partner is often the first clue of possible infection. Invasion into the peritoneal cavity usually occurs by the second or third menstrual period, after which inflammatory pelvic symptoms may develop. Chronic undetected infection may lead to septicemia, heart disease, gonococcal arthritis, or other debilitating conditions.
	  c. Newborn: conjunctivitis or other signs of inflammation of mucous tissue. Prophylactic treatment of the eyes of all newborns is often required by law.
		1. Antibiotic treatment per MP.
		2. Obtain history of intimate contact during periods of contagion; refer to public health agency for appropriate follow-through.
		3. Counseling and guidance as indicated for emotional and social problems.

Table 6-2. Symptoms of commonly misused drugs and poisons*

Agent	Symptoms	Agent	Symptoms

Amphetamine	CNS stimulation with restlessness, apprehension, irritability, delirium, hallucinations, tremors, and convulsions, followed by profound depression
	Gastrointestinal distress
	Dilated pupils, dry mouth
		Ethyl alcohol —cont'd	Blood levels of 0.15%-0.3%—slurring of speech, definite visual impairment, muscular incoordination, sensory loss
			Blood levels of 0.3%-0.5%—marked muscular incoordination, sensory loss, blurred or double vision, approaching stupor
			At 5% concentration—coma, slowed and labored respiration, decreased reflexes, and sensory loss; death can occur
			Gastrointestinal manifestations—one or more of the following:
			  Anorexia
			  Intermittent vomiting
			  Abdominal pain
			  Constipation
			CNS manifestations—one or more of the following:
			  Irritability
			  Drowsiness
			  Persistent vomiting
			  Incoordination
			  Convulsions
			  Coma
			  Weakness or paralysis
			  Hypertension
			  Papilledema and/or optic atrophy
			  Paralysis of one or more cranial nerves
			  Elevated cerebrospinal fluid protein content
			  Cerebrospinal fluid plocytosis
			  Elevated cerebrospinal fluid pressure
			Hematologic manifestations—one or more of the following:
			  Hypochromic microcytic anemia
			  Significant degree of basophilic stippling of red blood cells
			  75%-100% red fluorescence in erythrocytes examined under ultraviolet light
			  Radiologic density at metaphyses of long bones

Antihistamines	CNS depression (children may be stimulated) Atropinelike symptoms, dryness in mouth, fixed dilated pupils, flushing Gastrointestinal distress		
Aspirin	Gastrointestinal distress Hyperventilation Hyperpyrexia Hypoprothrombinemia Metabolic acidosis Hypoglycemia		
Barbiturates	Respiratory center depression with slow, shallow breathing; cyanosis often present Circulatory depression and shock due to depression of the vasomotor center, as well as direct action on smooth muscle in blood vessel wall Water loss from skin and lungs; decrease in urine output; electrolytes variable		
Chloral hydrate	CNS depression Cardiovascular depression Gastrointestinal distress Banana odor and blanching of lips "Knockout drops" are mixture of chloral and alcohol, producing potent depressant effect Caustic effects with esophagitis (stricture) and gastritis		
Codeine	CNS depression with muscular twitching and convulsions Weakness, disturbed vision, miosis, dyspnea Respiratory depression, collapse, coma		
Ethyl alcohol	CNS depression Blood levels of 0.05%-0.15%—slight muscular incoordination and visual impairment and slowing of reaction time	Marijuana	Exhiliration, euphoria, talkative, conjunctivitis, dryness of mouth Later quiet, drowsy, sleepy

*Adapted from Arena, J. M.: Poisoning and its treatment, Table 16-2. In Shirkey, H. C., editor: Pediatric therapy, ed. 5, St. Louis, 1975, The C. V. Mosby Co.

Continued.

Table 6-2. Symptoms of commonly misused drugs and poisons—cont'd

Agent	Symptoms	Agent	Symptoms
Marijuana —cont'd	Chronic effects are tremors, anorexia, pallor, weakness, mental deterioration, with reduction of will power and concentration Users have odor of burnt rope on person or clothing	Nicotine	CNS stimulation followed by depression; clonic convulsions, followed by collapse and respiratory failure Gastrointestinal distress, severe Caustic effects on mouth, throat, esophagus, stomach

Meprobamate	CNS depression
	Respiratory and cardiovascular collapse
	Stupor, coma, hypotension, miosis, loss of reflexes
		Parathion (phosphate ester insecticides)	Nicotinic effects
			  Incoordination
			  Fasciculation
			  Paralysis
			Muscarine effects
			  Miosis
			  Sweating, salivation, tearing
			  Pulmonary edema
			  Bradycardia and hypertension
			  Abdominal cramps, vomiting, diarrhea

Morphine	Profound CNS depression from above downward and stimulation from below upward
	Stupor, coma, miosis, slow and shallow respiration, cyanosis, tremors, convulsions
	Severe retching and nausea
			Effects
			  Apathy
			  Convulsions
			  Coma

CHAPTER 7

Sexual function
and family planning

The adolescent individual needs to have a great deal of support and help with the changes of puberty and the onset of reproductive function. Intellectual knowledge of male and female reproduction and sexual functions should be obtained during later childhood, but assuming that this has been the case may leave a great gap of understanding between the health care worker and the child. In a tactful and unobtrusive manner, the child's knowledge of sexual functioning for both sexes should be estimated, and offers to provide a further explanation and clarification may be made as appropriate. Young people may have questions that they are afraid to ask, and experience in working with young adolescents helps in developing an acceptable approach to dealing with their concerns.

Most adolescents are able to discuss their concerns only when their parents are not present, but the presence of a friend may enhance the discussion. Girls tend to be concerned about adequacy of development of their breasts, menstrual problems, and social relationships with boys. For girls, sexual feelings are diffuse, are not centered on genital function, and tend to be very romanticized. Questions and concerns about pregnancy, both in relation to initiation through coitus and the conduct of pregnancy through labor and delivery, begin to emerge as adolescence progresses. Concerns about homo-

sexual feelings or experiences and masturbation are also common among girls.

Boys are primarily concerned about the development of their genital organs and secondary signs of masculinity and about specific aspects of coitus. Because their sexual arousal is centered in the genital area and leads directly to desire for relief of tension through orgasm, boys experience a relatively early concern for this particular function of the body. In relation to this, they are curious and concerned about the female body and its function, but questions and concern about pregnancy and the initiation of pregnancy are not prominent. The urge to masturbate may be quite significant for the boy, and his feelings of acceptability or unacceptability of this practice may present a very important concern. The young person may have gross misunderstandings in relation to masturbation. Desire for social contact with girls is a prominent concern but is not romanticized as for girls, and permanent mate-seeking is not as prominent an urge for boys.

Intellectual understanding before puberty or during puberty may not alleviate the emotional concerns and problems encountered during adolescence in relation to sexual functioning. These matters are crowded into the individual's thinking, living, and behaving, and they become central to all that he or she does at certain

103

points in adolescent development. These concerns are not easily discussed, and often young people must approach the subject themselves before successful health guidance can be attempted. This is one instance where printed material is almost always received and read carefully; young people find the subject irresistible, and they eagerly seek all information and written discussion that they can possibly find. Materials that are directed to their level of interest and that include a discussion of all the physical and emotional concerns that they might be experiencing are particularly helpful. Young people may be given the opportunity to discuss what they are given to read when they are ready, but they may indicate their desire and readiness to talk in a very subtle manner. The necessity for skill in working with adolescents cannot be overemphasized for the health care worker who seeks to develop the ability to recognize and respond to their unique concerns.

It may be helpful to ask to see the material that the young person reads. He or she may feel embarrassed to share this with a health care worker, either because of the source of the material or because the material is considered undesirable by society. However, knowing the type of literature that young people are finding on their own is helpful in identifying some of their misunderstandings and inaccurate perceptions related to sexual functioning.

FAMILY PLANNING

An important aspect of health care in relation to newly acquired reproductive capacity is information and counseling regarding family planning, or contraception. All adolescents should become thoroughly acquainted with the methods available. As a professional health care worker, moral judgment must be laid aside in counseling with individual teenagers and in recognizing a very real health need that a young person may have in this regard. Both boys and girls should understand each of the methods of contraception, and they should know where to obtain help and advice when they need it. The community and the family of an individual teenager may have reservations or strong objections to the availability of such information, and the impact of these preferences should be fully

understood and respected. However, individual teenagers have the right and privilege of obtaining information and of making an autonomous choice in the matter as long as they understand the consequences of their choice and are willing to assume responsibility for it. They can be encouraged to know and understand the teachings of their culture, family, and religion in regard to family planning and to make their own choice based on each aspect of their situation. Although they are limited in regard to legal rights and responsibilities by being identified as a minor in American society, they retain personal rights that must be advocated if health care needs are adequately met.

Contraception

The *rhythm method* of contraception involves identification of the time of ovulation during the female cycle and abstinence from coitus during the normal life span of sperm before ovulation and for the life span of the ovum after ovulation. Ordinarily, ovulation occurs 14 days before the last day of a uterine cycle, but variation in timing of ovulation from cycle to cycle and from individual to individual makes exact prediction of this event difficult. To use the rhythm method with some assurance the woman's cycle must be fairly regular from month to month.

An estimate of the usual time of ovulation is made by identifying the longest and the shortest cycle that occur over a period of time and then estimating the range of time when fertilization is possible. The days of abstinence from coitus for all future cycles are then estimated until either a shorter or a longer cycle is experienced, and then the days of abstinence are reestimated. The first day of abstinence is calculated by subtracting 18 from the length of the shortest cycle. The figure 18 is derived by adding 2 days of sperm life and 2 days for possible variation of the time of ovulation to 14, the theoretical day of ovulation counting backward. The last day of abstinence is determined by subtracting 11 from the longest cycle. The figure 11 is derived from subtracting 2 days for possible variation in time of ovulation and 1 day for the life span of the ovum from 14, the theoretical day of ovulation. This gives the widest theoretical range during which fertilization might occur. Thus, if a woman records her shortest cycle as being 23 days and her longest as being 28, she must abstain from coitus from the fifth through the seventeenth day of all future cycles.

Reliability of the rhythm method may be increased for some women by also using temperature estimates of the time of ovulation. Ovulation is presumed to occur when basal awakening body temperature is the lowest, and the time of fertilizability of the ovum is considered to be past when the temperature has elevated at least 0.5° F and continues this elevation for at least 72 hours. Thus abstinence may begin as estimated by the 18-11 methods, but the time of again engaging in sexual relations may be determined by the basal body temperature.

The rhythm method is reported to have a failure rate of 14% to 40% in people using it for a year, as defined by the number of pregnancies that occur while this method of contraception is being used. Since the risk of becoming pregnant when no control method is used is 80%, the rhythm method of control has some value, but the pregnancy risk must be understood. When the basal body temperature determination is combined with the rhythm method, the failure rate is significantly lowered.

The *diaphragm* is a small rubber dome molded onto a circular rim that is fitted over the cervical os to occlude the entry of sperm into the uterus. It is used in combination with a spermicidal cream or jelly and thus provides both a mechanical and chemical barrier. The device must be obtained from a health care agency and is not available in drug stores, since it must be fitted to the size of the woman's cervix. Use of the diaphragm requires some amount of manipulation, which is troublesome and inconvenient, and the failure rate is about 12%. However, because of its safety its use has become more popular.

The *condom* is also used to provide a mechanical barrier to the entry of sperm into the uterus. This method of contraception is probably attempted by most young teenage boys, and the everyday peer-group sources of sex information usually include some description of the use of condoms. They are not considered popular for most adults because of the decrease in sensation

for the man and the inability of the woman to feel ejaculation, but they are undoubtedly popular because of their wide availability in drug stores, and large numbers are sold annually. Condoms are recommended as a protection against venereal disease, but because only a small skin area is covered by the sheath, protection is limited. The sheaths are made of rubber or plastic material and are usually supplied in a rolled form ready to be unrolled onto the erect penis. A small portion of the sheath is left at the end as a receptacle for the seminal fluid. The failure rate with proper usage is about 18%.

Chemical contraceptives are also readily available in drug stores without prescription. They come in the form of creams, jellies, and foams, and their use is relatively simple and inexpensive. However, they must be applied just before coitus, and they involve some decrease in sensation and some inconvenience because of messiness. The failure rate is high, averaging about 30%; thus they are usually recommended in combination with another method of control.

The *oral contraceptive pill* first became available to women in the United States in 1960, and because of hazards and potential complications it has become a less popular form of contraceptive control. The exact action of each form of the pill varies, but the basic principle is the prevention of ovulation by chemically altering the usual endocine cycle. Most forms of the pill contain estrogen, which raises the circulating level of this hormone early in the menstrual cycle. Since high levels of estrogen prevent the release of FSH by the pituitary gland, ovarian follicles are not stimulated to mature, and ovulation is prevented. When progesterone is added to the estrogen preparation, the endometrium of the uterus is stimulated to develop as during a normal cycle, and withdrawal of the pill causes a menstrual period to occur, simulating the normal ovulatory cycle.

The pill has certain bothersome side effects for some women, including weight gain, nausea, and breast tenderness simulating a pregnant state. Other side effects include headache, regression of gum tissue around the teeth, eye complications, and blood pressure increase. The serious side effects that have been substantiated are the risk of thromboembolic disease, hypertension, and cancer. Thus the pill is never recommended for a woman who has a known prior experience with blood clotting problems or who has a strong family history of cancer or heart disease. The risk of serious illness or death from the use of the pill is less than that expected from normal pregnancy and childbirth, and the pill is generally considered to be a safe, convenient, and reliable form of contraception for brief periods of time. The woman who uses the pill enhances the safety of its use by having regular evaluations of her progress and condition supervised by a health care professional, and most physicians and dispensing agents require that the woman seek annual health care before the prescription for the drug is renewed.

Use of the pill requires that the woman take 20 pills on consecutive days beginning with the fifth day of each cycle. If a pill is forgotten, it is taken as soon as the error is discovered. If the time span exceeds 12 hours after the usual time of taking the pill, another form of contraception should be used for the remainder of the cycle. Women who find remembering to take the pill daily difficult or impossible should use another form of contraception. The failure rate of the pill when it is used properly is about 0.6%. Most instances of failure result from forgetting to take the pill regularly.

The *intrauterine device (IUD)* is a small plastic or metal device that is placed in the uterus and remains indefinitely. It prevents pregnancy by interfering with implantation of the fertilized ovum. The exact mechanism by which this interference occurs is not known, but it appears that the device may affect the timing of when the fertilized egg reaches the endometrium, or it may cause the accumulation of cytotoxic compounds within the uterus that interfere with implantation. The most common side effects of the IUD are increased menstrual flow and associated pain, particularly in the early months after insertion. Serious risks include perforation of the uterine wall during insertion and transmission of infection into the uterus and abdominal cavity. These risks may be significantly decreased with appropriate insertion techniques.

Risk of pregnancy with the IUD has been decreased in recent years with improved devices to as low as 1.1% to 3%. Spontaneous expulsion of the device may occur, and a string is left on most devices, hanging below the level of the cervix so that the woman may determine the continued placement of the device.

For various reasons, *other methods* of contraception might be considered or attempted by young people, such as douches, coitus interruptus, or homemade occlusive devices. These attempts and experimentations need to be understood by the health care worker, and the young person needs assistance in realizing the problems involved and the greatly increased risk of failure. Breast-feeding, often thought to prevent ovulation, is not a reliable means of contraception beyond the sixth week after childbirth. Ovulation can occur before postpartum menstrual flow appears, and the young mother needs to consider beginning some form of family planning if she wishes to delay the next pregnancy.

Sterilization

The vasectomy is the most common surgical procedure used to render a man incapable of producing a pregnancy. The sperm duct is severed from each testicle, making it impossible for the sperm to pass from the testes into the urethra. It has no known effect on the male hormones, the testes, or the ability to have intercourse. It is a minor procedure and is often done in the physician's office.

The failure rate is low, and to assure the success of the procedure the man's semen is examined for the presence of sperm 6 to 8 weeks after the procedure is completed. The man and wife should understand that the procedure is probably irreversible. Most young men are not interested in this particular form of family planning but may consider it when they do not wish to have additional children or when a genetic problem has been detected that leads to serious problems for the family.

Sterilization for women includes abdominal or vaginal surgical procedures that range from removal of one or more of the reproductive organs to ligation of the tubes. These procedures involve a greater surgical risk and are most often performed in a hospital setting. The effects are irreversible. When a mother feels that she definitely does not wish to bear additional children, or when childbearing presents a serious risk to her or her family, she may consider such a step regardless of age. Sterilization can be accomplished immediately after delivery with a minimal amount of trauma, and for this reason counseling is directed to accomplishing this procedure at this particular time when such is known to be desirable. As with a vasectomy, surgical sterilization for the woman does not interfere with sexual function or enjoyment.

Abortion

When contraception fails or is not used and an unwanted pregnancy occurs, the problems for the adolescent girl are complex. Termination of pregnancy by means of abortion is mentioned here because of the growing use of this approach as a method of birth control in the United States. This has been the chief means of population control in the world for many centuries, and the illegal use of this procedure has created health problems for many years in the United States. Information regarding legal abortion is still relatively difficult for young people to obtain in most American cities, and social and legal aspects of the question remain extremely controversial. Abortion is condemned on philosophical, religious, social, and political grounds that require individual evaluation and personal judgments. Fears of physical or psychologic harm resulting to the woman are common, even though scientific evidence is lacking that untoward effects occur when a sound, acceptable method is used.

Abortion is most safely and efficiently accomplished before the end of the twelfth week of pregnancy. Local anesthesia may be used, and abortion is accomplished wither with dilation and curettage (D and C) or with vacuum or suction aspiration of the uterine lining. The procedure may be done without hospitalization. If abortion is required after the end of the first trimester, hospitalization is required and the surgical and medical procedures required are conducted under very close supervision.

CHAPTER 8

Guidelines to nutritional assessment*

Nutritional assessment of the child is one of the most important aspects of health care. To accomplish this aspect of assessment adequately, knowledge and understanding of cultural influences on the family, foods and their nutritional value, historically significant food fads, and economic factors influencing food habits need to be integrated with the information that is obtained about a particular child's nutrition.

Tables 8-1 and 8-2 present a summary of comprehensive nutritional assessment for infants and children. As reflected in these tables, each level of assessment requires a dietary history, a health and socioeconomic history, clinical evaluation of the child, and laboratory evaluations of blood and urine. The minimal level of nutritional assessment should be completed for every child at regular intervals during infancy, early childhood, later childhood, and adolescence. If any deficiencies are detected, midlevel or in-depth level assessment may be required using the resources of all members of the health care team, including physician, social worker, and nutritionist.

A diet history provides a basis for beginning detailed evaluation of a child's nutrition. An accurate accounting of foods eaten in a representative 24-hour period can provide basic information about the usual food habits of a child and his or her family. The health care worker relates this information to the general requirements of the four basic food groups, described on pp. 116 and 117. This information is also correlated with physical findings, such as height, weight, hematocrit, condition of the skin and teeth, and behavioral performance.

The two predominant nutrition-related problems of American society are (1) iron-deficiency anemia and (2) overweight and obesity. To combat the problem of iron-deficiency anemia the health assessment always includes regular monitoring of the hemoglobin or hematocrit, combined with knowledge of the child's usual intake of foods containing an adequate source of iron. Recommendations to provide a source of iron intake for all infants in the form of iron-fortified milk resulted in the provision of such formulas at no additional cost to the consumer. When iron-fortified milk is no longer a component of the child's diet, obtaining adequate food sources of iron becomes a very important economic issue and often requires special counseling and guidance for the young family.

The problem of obesity is ideally controlled during infancy, since obesity during infancy

*Prepared in consultation with Barbara Prater, R.D., M.S.

appears to be significantly related to problems of obesity during later childhood and adulthood. There are varying approaches that might be useful in helping the infant, child, or family toward controlling obesity, but the task is often difficult and discouraging. However, several principles of management appear to be significant in helping children and families prevent, control, or treat the problems related to being overweight.

1. Attempts to help only one member of a family are rarely successful. If only one member is overweight (even if this member is an infant), the problem cannot be isolated as being one of this individual alone. The entire family needs to understand the food habits that might be related to this individual's potential or real problem, and they must make appropriate adjustments in food habits on behalf of this individual. For example, if a family tends to celebrate daily events and enjoyments through the intake of food (often high calorie–low nutrition value food), this habit may be a significant contributor to the individual's problem. Even though other members of the family do not suffer the side effects of overweight, it is not reasonable to require only one person to change his eating habits. The temptation of cake and ice cream desserts every evening must be removed entirely!

2. Although calories may be calculated in detail to achieve some degree of calorie control, it may be most useful to begin by identifying the sources of "empty" calories and attempting to decrease or eliminate these from the diet. This approach is also useful in the prevention of obesity during infancy. Dessert foods, prepared baby food, adult foods that contain high concentrations of sugars and starch, snack foods, and sugar-containing beverages can be eliminated and substituted with foods of higher nutritional value and/or relatively less caloric value. *Note:* Infants and young children should not be placed on a diet that uses skim milk, even if there is a serious obesity problem. The essential fatty acids in whole milk are known to be crucial for adequate growth and development of healthy tissue, and calorie controls should be executed by altering other sources of excessive caloric intake, *not* milk.

3. Cultural and individual food preferences and habits will persist. Any attempts to help a family change food habits must be made within the context of the food preferences of the culture and of the individual family members.

4. Physical exercise is as intimately related to weight control as is food intake. In some instances it may be more important for a child to change his activity patterns than to alter his food habits. As with food habits, the entire family may need to become involved in helping a child to find pleasure and satisfaction from a different pattern of physical activity.

5. Adequate nutrition and caloric intake are essential during childhood and adolescence. "Crash" diets attempted by older children and adolescents may interfere with the requirements for maintenance of adequate growth and development. Attempts to seriously limit caloric intake should be carefully supervised by a physician. A diet that maintains weight while the child or adolescent continues to grow may be sufficient.

6. Obesity is rarely an isolated problem. There are often underlying factors that contribute to the excessive weight condition. Needs for attention, use of food as a behavioral reward, overprotection by parents, and insecurity have all been associated with the development of obesity. Certainly the causes are many and complex. Without seeking the analysis of causes of the problem, the health care worker may help the child and his family to develop basic knowledge of nutrition and foods, exercise, and overall healthy development and daily living. Realistic expectations for body size and build, appearance, behavioral performance, achievement in school and in life, or social success may be important issues to consider at the beginning. In some instances it may be more appropriate to help a young person develop a realistic and positive self-concept than to be concerned specifically about his obesity.

Finally, adequate nutrition counseling requires a substantial knowledge of the composition of foods and food products, which is usually beyond the scope of knowledge of most health care workers. When a specific nutrition problem is identified, dietary and nutrition specialists' assistance is most often indicated. The

Diet Record

Week of _____

Name _____

Food Groups to Include	Amounts to Include	Amounts of Food Actually Eaten (measured in household measurements)							Comments
		Mon.	Tues.	Wed.	Thurs.	Fri.	Sat.	Sun.	
1. Milk and Milk Products									
2. Meat and Meat Substitutes									
3. Vegetables									
4. Fruits									
5. Bread and Cereals									
6. Other									

Instructions:

1. Record the amounts of the listed food groups that you eat each day in the spaces provided.
2. Keep this sheet with you daily so that all foods can be recorded when they are eaten.
3. Use household measurements such as ½ cup, 1 tablespoon, 1 teaspoon, etc., to record the amounts of food.
4. Record all foods eaten.

Fig. 8-1. Sample of guideline for taking nutritional assessment.

Table 8-1. Levels of nutritional assessment for infants and children*

Level of approach†	History		Clinical evaluation	Laboratory evaluation
	Dietary	Medical and socioeconomic		
		BIRTH TO 24 MONTHS		
Minimal level	1. Source of iron 2. Vitamin supplement 3. Milk intake (type and amount)	1. Birth weight 2. Length of gestation 3. Serious or chronic illness 4. Use of medicines	1. Body weight and length 2. Gross defects	1. Hematocrit 2. Hemoglobin 3. Urine protein and sugar

Midlevel	1. Semi-quantitative
	  a. Iron-cereal, meat, egg yolks, supplement
	  b. Energy nutrients
	  c. Micronutrients—calcium, niacin, riboflavin, vitamin C
	  d. Protein
	2. Food intolerances
	3. Baby foods—processed commercially; home cooked
		1. Family history:
		Diabetes
		Tuberculosis
		2. Maternal:
		Height
		Prenatal care
		3. Infant:
		Immunizations
		Tuberculin test
			1. Head circumference
			2. Skin color, pallor, turgor
			3. Subcutaneous tissue paucity, excess
				1. RBC morphology
				2. Serum iron
				3. Total iron binding capacity
				4. Sickle cell testing

In-depth level	1. Quantitative 24-hour recall 2. Dietary history	1. Prenatal details 2. Complications of delivery 3. Regular health supervision	1. Cranial bossing 2. Epiphyseal enlargement 3. Costochondral beading 4. Ecchymoses	Same as above, plus vitamin and appropriate enzyme assays; protein and amino acids; hydroxyproline, etc., should be available
		FOR AGES 2 TO 5 YEARS		
	Determine amount of intake	Probe about pica Medications	Add height at all levels Add arm circumference at all levels Add triceps skinfolds at in-depth level	Add serum lead at midlevel Add serum micronutrients (vitamins A, C, folate, etc.) at in-depth level
		FOR AGES 6 TO 12 YEARS		
	Probe about snack foods Determine whether salt intake is excessive	Ask about medications taken; drug abuse	Add blood pressure at midlevel Add description of changes in tongue, skin, eyes for in-depth level	All of above plus BUN

*From Christakis, G., editor: Nutritional assessment in health programs, Am. J. Public Health [Suppl] **63**:1-82, Nov. 1973.
†It is understood that what is included at a minimal level would also be included or represented at successively more sophisticated levels of approach. However, it may be entirely appropriate to use a minimal level of approach to clinical evaluations and a maximal approach to laboratory evaluations.

tables contained in the following pages are provided as a beginning resource for initial evaluation of many problems that might be identified. For example, the daily dietary allowances are included to serve as a general reference in cursory evaluation of the diet of an infant or a family. To most completely utilize this information, however, one must know the exact nutritional content of foods that are eaten. General values for various foods may be estimated by reports on packages or in resources containing average food values for commonly ingested foods; but specific values are not easily determined and require special advanced nutrition knowledge.

Table 8-2. Levels of nutritional assessment for adolescents*

Levels of approach	History		Clinical evaluation	Laboratory evaluation
	Dietary	**Medical and socioeconomic**		
Minimal level	1. Frequency of use of food groups 2. Habits-patterns 3. Snacks 4. Socioeconomic status	1. Previous diseases and allergies 2. Abbreviated system review 3. Family history	1. Height 2. Weight	1. Urine, protein, and sugar 2. Hemoglobin
Midlevel	1. Above 2. Qualitative estimate 3. 24-hour recall	1. Above in more detail	1. Above 2. Arm circumference 3. Skinfold thickness 4. External appearance	1. Above 2. Blood taken by vein for albumin (serum), serum iron and TIBC; vitamins A and beta carotene; RBC indices; blood urea nitrogen (BUN); cholesterol; zinc
In-depth level	1. Above 2. Quantitative estimate by recall (3-7 days)	1. Above	1. Above 2. Per ICNND Manual 3. X-ray of wrist and bone density	1. Above 2. Blood tests: folate and vitamin C; alkaline phosphatase; RBC transketolase; RBC glutathione; lipids 3. Urine: creatinine; nitrogen; zinc; thiamine; riboflavin; loading tests (xanthurenic acid/FIGLU) 4. Hair root: DNA; protein; zinc, other metals

*From Christakis, G., editor: Nutritional assessment in health programs, Am. J. Public Health [Suppl] **63:**1-82, Nov. 1973.

Table 8-3. Calorie control guideline for girls*†

Age	10-12 years	12-14 years	14-16 years	16-18 years
Suggested calories per pound per day	29 calories	24 calories	21 calories	19 calories
Average height	56 inches	61 inches	62 inches	63 inches
Average weight	77 pounds	97 pounds	114 pounds	119 pounds
Total calories required/day	2,250	2,300	2,400	2,300

*From Leverton, R.: A girl and her figure. Reprinted by permission. Available from the National Dairy Council, Chicago, Ill., 60606.
†*Note:* Reference to a complete caloric and nutritional content of food resource is needed to aid the child in planning a dietary regimen.

Table 8-4. Calorie control guidelines for boys*†

Age	9-12 years	12-15 years	15-18 years
Suggested calories per pound per day	33 calories	31 calories	25 calories
Average height	55 inches	61 inches	68 inches
Average weight	72 pounds	98 pounds	134 pounds
Total calories required/day	2,400	3,000	3,400

*From Gregg, W. H.: A boy and his physique. Reprinted by permission. Available from the National Dairy Council, Chicago, Ill., 60606.
†*Note:* Reference to a complete caloric and nutritional content of food resource is needed to aid the child in planning a dietary regimen.

Table 8-5. Food and Nutrition Board, National Academy of Sciences—National Research Council Recommended Daily Dietary Allowances,[1] revised 1974 (designed for the maintenance of good nutrition of practically all healthy people in the U.S.A.)

	Age (years)	Weight		Height		Energy (kcal)[2]	Protein (g)	Fat-soluble vitamins			
								Vitamin A activity		Vitamin D (IU)	Vitamin E activity[4] (IU)
		kg	lb	cm	in			RE[3]	IU		
Infants	0.0-0.5	6	14	60	24	kg × 117	kg × 2.2	420[7]	1,400	400	4
	0.5-1.0	9	20	71	28	kg × 108	kg × 2.0	400	2,000	400	5
Children	1-3	13	28	86	34	1,300	23	400	2,000	400	7
	4-6	20	44	110	44	1,800	30	500	2,500	400	9
	7-10	30	66	135	54	2,400	36	700	3,300	400	10
Males	11-14	44	97	158	63	2,800	44	1,000	5,000	400	12
	15-18	61	134	172	69	3,000	54	1,000	5,000	400	15
	19-22	67	147	172	69	3,000	52	1,000	5,000	400	15
	23-50	70	154	172	69	2,700	56	1,000	5,000		15
	51+	70	154	172	69	2,400	56	1,000	5,000		15
Females	11-14	44	97	155	62	2,400	44	800	4,000	400	12
	15-18	54	119	162	65	2,100	48	800	4,000	400	12
	19-22	58	128	162	65	2,100	46	800	4,000	400	12
	23-50	58	128	162	65	2,000	46	800	4,000		12
	51+	58	128	162	65	1,800	46	800	4,000		12
Pregnant						+300	+30	1,000	5,000	400	15
Lactating						+500	+20	1,200	6,000	400	15

[1]The allowances are intended to provide for individual variations among most normal persons as they live in the United States under usual environmental stresses. Diets should be based on a variety of common foods in order to provide other nutrients for which human requirements have been less well defined.
[2]Kilojoules (KJ) = 4.2 × kcal.
[3]Retinol equivalents.
[4]Total vitamin E activity, estimated to be 80% as α-tocopherol and 20% other tocopherols.

Water-soluble vitamins							Minerals					
Ascorbic acid (mg)	Folacin[5] (μg)	Niacin[6] (mg)	Riboflavin (mg)	Thiamin (mg)	Vitamin B_6 (mg)	Vitamin B_{12} (μg)	Calcium (mg)	Phosphorus (mg)	Iodine (μg)	Iron (mg)	Magnesium (mg)	Zinc (mg)
35	50	5	0.4	0.3	0.3	0.3	360	240	35	10	60	3
35	50	8	0.6	0.5	0.4	0.3	540	400	45	15	70	5
40	100	9	0.8	0.7	0.6	1.0	800	800	60	15	150	10
40	200	12	1.1	0.9	0.9	1.5	800	800	80	10	200	10
40	300	16	1.2	1.2	1.2	2.0	800	800	110	10	250	10
45	400	18	1.5	1.4	1.6	3.0	1,200	1,200	130	18	350	15
45	400	20	1.8	1.5	1.8	3.0	1,200	1,200	150	18	400	15
45	400	20	1.8	1.5	2.0	3.0	800	800	140	10	350	15
45	400	18	1.6	1.4	2.0	3.0	800	800	130	10	350	15
45	400	16	1.5	1.2	2.0	3.0	800	800	110	10	350	15
45	400	16	1.3	1.2	1.6	3.0	1,200	1,200	115	18	300	15
45	400	14	1.4	1.1	2.0	3.0	1,200	1,200	115	18	300	15
45	400	14	1.4	1.1	2.0	3.0	800	800	100	18	300	15
45	400	13	1.2	1.0	2.0	3.0	800	800	100	18	300	15
45	400	12	1.1	1.0	2.0	3.0	800	800	80	10	300	15
60	800	+2	+0.3	+0.3	2.5	4.0	1,200	1,200	125	18+[8]	450	20
80	600	+4	+0.5	+0.3	2.5	4.0	1,200	1,200	150	18	450	25

[5]The folacin allowances refer to dietary sources as determined by *Lactobacillis casei* assay. Pure forms of folacin may be effective in doses less than one fourth of the RDA.

[6]Although allowances are expressed as niacin, it is recognized that on the average 1 mg of niacin is derived from each 60 mg of dietary tryptophan.

[7]Assumed to be all as retinol in milk during the first 6 months of life. All subsequent intakes are assumed to be one half as retinol and one half as β-carotene when calculated from international units. As retinol equivalents, three fourths are as retinol and one fourth as β-carotene.

[8]This increased requirement cannot be met by ordinary diets; therefore, the use of supplemental iron is recommended.

GUIDE TO GOOD EATING*

A recommended daily pattern

The recommended daily pattern provides the foundation for a nutritious, healthful diet.

The recommended servings from the Four Food Groups for adults supply about 1,200 calories. The chart below gives recommendations for the number and size of servings for several categories of people.

Food group	Recommended number of servings

Milk
 1 cup milk, yogurt, OR
 Calcium equivalent:
   1½ slices (1½ oz) cheddar
     cheese†
   1 cup pudding
   1¾ cups ice cream
   2 cups cottage cheese†
	Child: 3
	 Teenager: 4
	 Adult: 2
	 Pregnant woman: 4
	 Lactating woman: 4

Meat
 2 ounces cooked, lean meat,
  fish, poultry, OR
 Protein equivalent:
   2 eggs
   2 slices (2 oz) cheddar
     cheese†
   ½ cup cottage cheese†
   1 cup dried beans, peas
   4 tbsp peanut butter
	Child: 2
	 Teenager: 2
	 Adult: 2
	 Pregnant woman: 3
	 Lactating woman: 2

Fruit-vegetable
 ½ cup cooked or juice
 1 cup raw
 Portion commonly served
  such as a medium-size
  apple or banana
	Child: 4
	 Teenager: 4
	 Adult: 4
	 Pregnant woman: 4
	 Lactating woman: 4

Grain, whole grain, fortified, enriched 1 slice bread 1 cup ready-to-eat cereal ½ cup cooked cereal, pasta, grits	Child: 4 Teenager: 4 Adult: 4 Pregnant woman: 4 Lactating woman: 4

*Courtesy National Dairy Council, ed. 4, copyright 1977.
†Count cheese as serving of milk OR meat, not both simultaneously.
"Others" complement but do not replace foods from the Four Food Groups. Amounts should be determined by individual caloric needs.

Nutrients for health

Nutrient	Important sources of nutrient
Protein	Meat, poultry, fish Dried beans and peas Egg Cheese Milk
Carbohydrate	Cereal Potatoes Dried beans Corn Bread Sugar
Fat	Shortening, oil Butter, margarine Salad dressing Sausages
Vitamin A (retinol)	Liver Carrots Sweet potatoes Greens Butter, margarine
Vitamin C (ascorbic acid)	Broccoli Orange Grapefruit Papaya Mango Strawberries
Thiamin (B_1)	Lean pork Nuts Fortified cereal products
Riboflavin (B_2)	Liver Milk Yogurt Cottage cheese
Niacin	Liver Meat, poultry, fish Peanuts Fortified cereal products
Calcium	Milk, yogurt Cheese Sardines and salmon with bones Collard, kale, mustard, and turnip greens
Iron	Enriched farina Prune juice Liver Dried beans and peas Red meat

Nutrients are chemical substances obtained from foods during digestion. They are needed to build and maintain body cells, regulate body processes, and supply energy.

About 50 nutrients, including water, are needed daily for optimum health. If one obtains the proper amount of the 10 "leader" nutrients in the daily diet, the other 40 or so nutrients will likely be consumed in amounts sufficient to meet body needs.

One's diet should include a variety of foods because no *single* food supplies all the 50 nutrients, and because many nutrients work together.

When a nutrient is added or a nutritional claim is made, nutrition labeling regulations require listing the 10 leader nutrients on food packages. These nutrients appear in the chart below with food sources and some major physiologic functions.

Some major physiologic functions

Provide energy	Build and maintain body cells	Regulate body processes
Supplies 4 calories per gram.	Constitutes part of the structure of every cell, such as muscle, blood, and bone; supports growth and maintains healthy body cells.	Constitutes part of enzymes, some hormones and body fluids, and antibodies that increase resistance to infection.
Supplies 4 calories per gram. Major source of energy for central nervous system.	Supplies energy so protein can be used for growth and maintenance of body cells.	Unrefined products supply fiber—complex carbohydrates in fruits, vegetables, and whole grains—for regular elimination. Assists in fat utilization.
Supplies 9 calories per gram.	Constitutes part of the structure of every cell. Supplies essential fatty acids.	Provides and carries fat-soluble vitamins (A, D, E, and K).
	Assists formation and maintenance of skin and mucous membranes that line body cavities and tracts, such as nasal passages and intestinal tract, thus increasing resistance to infection.	Functions in visual processes and forms visual purple, thus promoting healthy eye tissues and eye adaptation in dim light.
	Forms cementing substances, such as collagen, that hold body cells together, thus strengthening blood vessels, hastening healing of wounds and bones, and increasing resistance to infection.	Aids utilization of iron.
Aids in utilization of energy.		Functions as part of a coenzyme to promote the utilization of carbohydrate. Promotes normal appetite. Contributes to normal functioning of nervous system.
Aids in utilization of energy.		Functions as part of a coenzyme in the production of energy within body cells. Promotes healthy skin, eyes, and clear vision.
Aids in utilization of energy.		Functions as part of a coenzyme in fat synthesis, tissue respiration, and utilization of carbohydrate. Promotes healthy skin, nerves, and digestive tract. Aids digestion and fosters normal appetite.
	Combines with other minerals within a protein framework to give structure and strength to bones and teeth.	Assists in blood clotting. Functions in normal muscle contraction and relaxation, and normal nerve transmission.
Aids in utilization of energy.	Combines with protein to form hemoglobin, the red substance in blood that carries oxygen to and carbon dioxide from the cells. Prevents nutritional anemia and its accompanying fatigue. Increases resistance to infection.	Functions as part of enzymes involved in tissue respiration.

Table 8-6. Composition and analysis of commercial formulas—nutrient values of 1 oz normal dilutions*

Name of formula and description	Composition	Calories	Carbo-hydrate (g)	Protein (g)	Fat (g)	Ca (g)	P (g)	Fe (g)	Vitamins					
									A (USP)	B_1 (mg)	B_2 (mg)	C (mg)	D (USP)	Niacin (mg)
Bakers formula: scientifically formulated to approximate the nutritional results of human milk	Skim milk, vegetable oils, lactose, dextrins, maltose, dextrose, vitamins and minerals	20	1.96	0.62	0.92	0.024	0.02	0.23		0.019	0.03	1.6	12.5	0.16
Bremil: powdered infant food	Skim milk, lactose, vegetable oils, vitamins and minerals	20	1.96	0.42	0.98	0.02	0.011	0.25	78	0.013	0.031	1.6	12.5	0.19
Carnalac: prepared evaporated milk formula	Evaporated milk, vitamins and minerals	20	2.30	0.67	0.75	0.002	0.017	0.019	40	0.0005	0.034	2.5	2.5	0.019
Enfamil: nearly identical to mother's milk	Skim milk, lactose, vegetable oils, soy lecithin, carrageenin, vitamins and minerals	20	1.96	0.42	1.0	0.018	0.014	0.044	50	0.013	0.019	1.6	12.5	0.125
Enfamil with iron: nearly identical to mother's milk with supplemental iron	Skim milk, lactose, vegetable oils, soy lecithin, carrageenin, vitamins and minerals	20	1.96	0.42	1.0	0.018	0.014	0.25	50	0.013	0.019	1.6	12.5	0.125
Isomil: soy isolate for use in milk allergies	Sucrose, corn syrup, soy protein isolate, corn oil, vitamins and minerals	20	1.9	0.56	0.73	0.022	0.016	0.38	78	0.013	0.019	1.6	12.5	†
Lofenalac: low phenylalanine food	Casein hydrolysate, corn oil, dextri-maltose, arrowroot starch, sucrose, amino acids, vitamins and minerals	20	2.38	—	0.76	0.028	0.02	0.42	47	0.014	0.056	0.94	12.5	0.125
Lamb base formula: special purpose food to use as a replacement for milk	Lamb hearts, dextrins, modified tapioca starch, vegetable oil, vitamins and minerals	20	2.21	0.67	0.67	0.02	0.016	0.23	47	0.008	0.03	1.4	12.5	0.16

Modilac: regular infant formula	Skim milk, dextrins, vegetable oil, vitamins and minerals	20	2.18	0.62	0.75	0.025	0.019	0.31	47	0.016	0.031	1.4	12.5	†
Mull-soy: hypoallergenic food for infants and children	Soy flour, soy oil, sucrose, dextrose, dextrins, vitamins and minerals	20	1.45	0.87	1.0	0.034	0.022	0.14	62.5	0.016	0.025	1.25	12.5	0.28
Nutramigen: protein hydrolysate formula	Sugar, casein, vegetable oil, arrowroot, vitamins and minerals	20	2.38	0.62	0.77	0.028	0.02	0.40	47	0.014	0.057	1.88	12.5	0.13
Probana: high protein formula with banana powder	Whole milk curd, skim milk powder, lactic acid, casein hydrolysate, banana powder, dextrose, vitamins and minerals	20	2.21	1.18	0.62	0.031	0.003	0.09	160	†	†	†	31	†
Prosobee: milk-free formula with soy isolate	Sugar, soy oil, soy protein isolate, corn syrup, vitamins and minerals	20	1.9	0.70	0.95	0.028	0.019	0.25	47	0.02	0.03	1.6	12.5	0.22
Similac 20: regular infant formula	Skim milk, lactose, vegetable oils, carrageenin, vitamins and minerals	20	1.96	0.50	1.00	0.022	0.016	‡	78	0.02	0.03	1.6	12.5	†
Similac 20 with iron: regular infant formula	Skim milk, lactose, vegetable oils, carrageenin, vitamins and minerals	20	1.96	0.50	1.00	0.22	0.016	0.38	78	0.02	0.03	1.6	12.5	†
SMA-26: infant formula patterned after human milk in nutritional balance	Skim milk, demineralized whey, lactose, oleo, vegetable oils, carrageenin, vitamins and minerals	20	2.0	0.42	1.0	0.012	0.009	0.27	78	0.02	0.03	1.6	12.5	0.16
Gerber's meat base formula (undiluted): special purpose food to use as a replacement for milk	Beef hearts, sugar, vegetable oils, modified tapioca starch, vitamins and minerals	43	2.77	1.9	2.1	0.075	0.05	1.15	115	0.038	0.10	31.	30.8	†

Continued.

*From Primary Children's Hospital diet manual, Salt Lake City, Utah, revised Oct. 1972.
†Undetermined amount.
‡Trace in ingredients.

Table 8-6. Composition and analysis of commercial formulas—nutrient values of 1 oz normal dilutions—cont'd

Name of formula and description	Composition	Calories	Carbo-hydrate (g)	Pro-tein (g)	Fat (g)	Ca (g)	P (g)	Fe (g)	Vitamins A (USP)	B₁ (mg)	B₂ (mg)	C (mg)	D (USP)	Niacin (mg)
Special milks and supplements														
Casec: protein preparation as a modifier for infant formula	Calcium caseinate powder	17/Tb		4/Tb	0.56	0.075/Tb	0.22							
Lactic acid milk: acidified whole milk 1 ounce undiluted	Whole milk and lactic acid	40/Tb	10.3/Tb	7.28/Tb	7.62/Tb	0.03/Tb	0.02/Tb	0.00008/Tb						
Lonalac: low sodium milk	Lactose, coconut oil, casein, vitamins and minerals	20	1.34	0.95	0.98	0.03	0.03	0.07	30	0.01	0.05			.03

Electrolyte replacements (all values per liter)	Composition	Cal	Na	K	Ca	Mg	Citrate	Dextrose	Sulfate	Chl	P	Lactate
Lytren: oral electrolyte formulation for replacement of fluid and electrolytes	Sodium citrate, potassium chloride, sodium bi-phosphate, citric acid, calcium lactate, sodium chloride, magnesium sulfate, dextrose, maltose, and dextrin	8	25 mEq	25 mEq	4 mEq	4 mEq	15 mEq	—	4 mEq	30 mEq	5 mEq	4 mEq
Pedialyte: oral electrolyte solution	Dextrose, sodium lactate, potassium chloride, calcium chloride, magnesium chloride, and sodium chloride	6	30 mEq	20 mEq	4 mEq	4 mEq	—	50 g	—	30 mEq	—	28 mEq

CHAPTER 9

Community and national resources

The following list of community and national resources is a compilation of some of the most widely available agencies and organizations providing specific assistance for families and professional health care workers. Each of the agencies listed gives both professional and consumer assistance, and families in need of special assistance may be referred to the agency directly. In most instances the address of the national organization is provided even though local branches exist throughout the United States and Canada. Often a local agency can be located through the telephone directory; if not, the national organizations can provide information concerning the nearest agency serving a given community. Brief comment is provided giving a summary of the specific services offered by each organization. For further information and a more detailed listing of various community resources, the reader is referred to the Encyclopedia of Associations, vol. I, National Organizations of the United States, Gale Research Book Tower, Detroit, Michigan.

ORGANIZATIONS FOR COMMUNITY, FAMILY, AND CHILD HEALTH PROMOTION

American Academy of Pediatrics
P.O. Box 1034
Evanston, Illinois 60204

Literature for families, parents, and professional health groups related to child health, illness, and welfare.

American Civil Liberties Union, Inc.
22 East 40th Street
New York, New York 10016

To protect free inquiry and expression, due process, fair trial and equality before the law, and so on by combating repressive legislation and the acts of officials in violation of civil liberties; to aid in the defense of cases in courts and to carry test cases to the higher courts.

American Dental Association, Inc.
211 East Chicago Avenue
Chicago, Illinois 60611

To improve oral and dental health services to the public by cultivating and promoting the art and science of dentistry through the following means: encouraging and providing for dental research; disseminating among the profession advanced scientific knowledge; elevating and sustaining the education of dentists in formal institutions of learning; and establishing devices that provide opportunities for continuing education after graduation.

American Institute of Family Relations
5287 Sunset Boulevard
Los Angeles, California 90027

Educational campaign through books, pamphlets, radio, television, newspapers, magazines, summer workshops in counseling, seminars, lectures, and a monthly bulletin. Trains teachers and counselors;

supplies materials to college and high school instructors, community executives, hospital personnel, and leaders in religious education for use in their classes.

American Medical Association
535 North Dearborn
Chicago, Illinois 60610

To promote the science and art of medicine, and to aid in the betterment of public health. Activities related to social work include those represented by the association's Department of Health Education and Department of Investigation (dealing especially with fraud and quackery in medicine).

American National Red Cross
17th and D Streets, N.W.
Washington, D.C. 20006

Service to the armed forces and their families; service to the veterans and their families; disaster services; blood services; health and community services.

American Public Health Association, Inc.
1015 18th Street, N.W.
Washington, D.C. 20036

To protect and promote public health by field surveys, publishing methods and manuals in program areas such as accident prevention, communicable diseases, and so on.

American Public Welfare Association
1155 16th Street, Suite 201
Washington, D.C. 20036

To assist in the development and maintenance of sound principles and effective administration of public welfare services; technical consultant and advisory services to the legislative and administrative authorities.

American School Health Association
Kent State University
Kent, Ohio 44240

Comprehensive and constructive school health programs including the teaching of health and health services and healthful school living.

American Women's Voluntary Services
135 East 65th Street
New York, New York 10021

To offer an opportunity to every woman to serve her country and her community loyally and efficiently without regard to creed, color, or age. Recruits, mobilizes, and trains women for all types of community service and places them where they may be a maximum assistance to give service to recognized local agencies.

Child Study Association of America
Wel Met, Inc.
50 Madison Avenue
New York, New York 10010

Provides parent education materials.

Child Welfare League of America
67 Irving Place
New York, New York 10003

To develop standards of service for the protection and care of children in their own homes or away from home through boarding home care, institutional care, adoption, day care, or homemaker service; and in community programs through the following means: cooperation with governmental departments of child welfare, publications, information exchange service, loan library and record forms, case record collection, general information and education in the field service consultation, and regional agencies.

Family Service Association of America
44 East 23rd Street
New York, New York 10010

Counseling and mental health services to families under stress; preventing family breakdown, promoting the development of family social work and wholesome family life through the following means: field service for family service agencies, assistance in development of qualified personnel in family casework, information and research on family life.

Food Distribution Division
Agricultural Marketing Service
U.S. Department of Agriculture
Washington, D.C. 20250

Administers the National School Lunch Program and Food Stamp Program.

Health Information Foundation
Graduate School of Business
The University of Chicago
Chicago, Illinois 60637

Contributes through social and economic research and through education toward the continual improvement of health services in the United States.

Its primary objectives are to assist in the distribution of health services to all segments of the population and to add knowledge that will facilitate payment for medical care.

Homebirth
89 Franklin Street, Suite 200
Boston, Massachusetts 02110

Provides information and instruction for preparation for birth at home, and assists couples in locating professional licensed attendants for home birth. Provides criteria and instructions for safe home delivery.

La Leche League International, Inc.
9616 Minneapolis Avenue
Franklin Park, Illinois 60131
Provides support for nursing mothers.

Maternity Center Association, Inc.
48 East 92nd Street
New York, New York 10028
To improve maternity care through the following means: teaching the public what adequate maternity care is and why it is necessary; training graduate nurses in midwifery; providing units in advanced maternity nursing for public health nurses and conducting refresher institutes in obstetrics for them; publishing handbooks on maternity care; providing motion pictures and film strips for nurses, expectant mothers and fathers, and high school and college students.

National Academy of Sciences
2101 Constitution Avenue, N.W.
Washington, D.C. 20418
Provides recommended dietary allowance and other nutrition resources.

National Alliance of Businessmen (NAB)
1730 K Street, N.W.
Washington, D.C. 20006
To find employment for disadvantaged people such as the poor, handicapped, and those who have been in prison.

National Association for the Advancement of Colored People
1790 Broadway
New York, New York 10019
To win full political, civil, and legal rights for colored citizens and to secure for them equality of opportunity.

National Association for the Education of Young Children
1834 Connecticut Avenue, N.W.
Washington, D.C. 20009
To provide an organization for the advancement of nursery education through meetings and publications and to facilitate operation with other agencies concerned with the education and well-being of young children.

National Committee on Employment of Youth of the National Child Labor Committee
145 East 32nd Street
New York, New York 10016
Concentrates on the problems of young people who are seeking suitable employment.

National Committee on Homemaker Services
67 Irving Place
New York, New York 10003
To promote improvement in the quality of homemaker services and to stimulate the extension of services under both voluntary and public auspices in communities throughout the country.

National Conference of Catholic Charities
1346 Connecticut Avenue, N.W.
Washington, D.C. 20036
Particular emphasis on service for children and youth; for example, foster care, counseling (unmarried parents), adoption services (statewide), short-term counseling to families and youth, emergency material assistance.

National Congress of American Indians
1430 K Street, N.W.
Washington, D.C. 20005
To secure to members of the Indian tribes and their descendants the rights and benefits to which they are entitled under the laws of the United States and the several states. To enlighten the public toward a better understanding of the Indian people; to preserve Indian cultural values; to seek an equitable adjustment of tribal affairs; to secure and to preserve rights under Indian treaties or agreements with the United States; and otherwise to promote the common welfare of the American Indians.

National Council on Family Relations
1219 University Avenue, S.E.
Minneapolis, Minnesota 55414
To provide opportunities for organized groups, agencies, members of allied professions, and individuals interested in family life to plan and act together voluntarily for the advancement of marriage and family life by means of consultation, conference, and cooperation on the goals, needs, and problems of marriage and family living.

National Dairy Council
300 North River Road
Rosemont, Illinois 60018
Provides nutrition literature and audiovisual educational aids including useful reviews of recent nutrition research in the *Dairy Council Digest*.

National Legal Aid and Defender Association
American Bar Center
Chicago, Illinois 60637
To promote and develop legal aid and defender work; to encourage the formation of new legal

aid and defender organizations wherever they may be needed.

National Organization for Women
425 13th Street, N.W., Suite 1001
Washington, D.C. 20004

Provides counseling and guidance for women in relation to personal development, job and career opportunities, child care, and political action.

National Safety Council
444 North Michigan Avenue
Chicago, Illinois 60611

To reduce the number and severity of all kinds of accidents at home, on the farm, at work, in the schools, and on the streets and highways.

Nutrition and Consumer-use Research
Agricultural Research Service
Department of Agriculture
Washington, D.C. 20250

Research organization conducting scientific studies of special concern to the home including food and nutrition, household economics, textiles and clothing, and housing and household equipment.

Parents Without Partners, Inc.
7910 Woodmont Avenue, Suite 1000
Washington, D.C. 20014

To develop and provide a broad comprehensive program for the enlightenment and guidance of parents without partners and their children on the special problems they encourter and for assistance on the various readjustments involved.

Planned Parenthood Federation of America, Inc.
810 Seventh Avenue
New York, New York 10019

To provide leadership for universal acceptance of family planning as an essential element of responsible family life through education, service, and research.

Play Schools Association, Inc.
111 East 59th Street
New York, New York 10022

A national voluntary agency serving school-age children and their parents directly and through affiliated organizations. It demonstrates, sets standards, and strengthens group-center play programs after school during the school year and all day during the summer

President's Council on Physical Fitness
Room 4830 GOA Building
411 G Street, N.W.
Washington, D.C. 20001

Promotes school health and physical fitness pro-grams in operation with existing educational and medical organizations, youth service groups, and state and local agencies.

Public Health Service
Department of Health, Education, and Welfare
Washington, D.C. 20203

Principal federal health agency; includes programs in the prevention and control of communicable and chronic diseases, occupational disease, mental health, and environmental health and sanitation, particularly water and air pollution control; hospital and medical facilities.

United Health Foundations, Inc.
2 East 103rd Street
New York, New York 10010

Coordinates research and health education activities of its members. Does the following programs: receives and allocates research funds; approves and certifies local research funds; develops health information and education materials; advises members on their health education; conducts demonstration programs in health education; acts as a national information clearinghouse for members; on request represents members in matters of mutual interest with public and voluntary health agencies, medical organizations, and other groups in the field of health.

ORGANIZATIONS FOR SPECIFIC HEALTH PROBLEMS

American Cancer Society, Inc.
777 Third Avenue
New York, New York 10017

Seeks the control of cancer through a three-point program of research, education, and service. Brings information about cancer to the lay public and current information on cancer detection and treatment to physicians. The service program goal is to aid in preventing deaths from cancer by supporting physicians' efforts to provide earlier and improved treatment of cancer and to bring greater comfort to cancer patients. Funds are secured through voluntary contributions from the public and from legacies.

American Child Guidance Foundation, Inc.
18 Tremont Street
Boston, Massachusetts 02100

To develop and maintain a continuing program to assist professional groups, agencies, organizations, clinics, university departments, and so on in the development and application of more effective means for the prevention and better control of childhood emotional and behavioral disorders.

American Diabetes Association, Inc.
1 West 48th Street
New York, New York 10020

To further general welfare through acquisition and dissemination of useful and accurate knowledge and information regarding diabetes mellitus; to undertake in the public interest such activities as will improve the physical welfare of persons having that disorder.

American Foundation for the Blind
15 West 16th Street
New York, New York 10011

Prevention and education programs; services for blind individuals and their families.

American Hearing Society, Inc.
919 18th Street, N.W.
Washington, D.C. 20006

To prevent deafness, preserve hearing, and rehabilitate the hard of hearing. Encourages nationwide audiometer testing of school children at regular intervals and follow-up as indicated.

American Heart Association, Inc.
44 East 23rd Street
New York, New York 10011

To support cardiovascular research and bring its benefits to the professional and lay public through community service and education programs; to coordinate efforts of physicians, nurses, social workers and others combating heart diseases; to inform the public of progress in the field and enlist support of the program through the annual Heart Fund campaign.

American Printing House for the Blind, Inc.
1839 Frankfort Avenue
Louisville, Kentucky 40206

Literature and appliances for the blind on a nonprofit basis.

Arthritis and Rheumatism Foundation
3400 Peachtree Road, N.E.
Atlanta, Georgia 30326

To provide special training in rheumatic diseases to more doctors; to increase the number of scientists investigating these diseases; to finance the development and enlargement of research, training, and treatment centers.

Association for the Aid of Crippled Children
345 East 46th Street
New York, New York 10017

Devoted to the prevention of crippling diseases and conditions and to improvement in the care of disabled children and youth and in their adjustment in society. Grants are made here and abroad to support research on prenatal life, perinatal mortality, and the social and emotional factors in disability. Conferences are conducted to stimulate communication and collaboration in rehabilitation and research and to open new areas of investigation. In conjunction with these aims, technical and popular materials are published, and consultation is provided to organizations and individuals professionally involved in the fields of the Association's interest.

Family Location Service, Inc.
33 West 60th Street
New York, New York 10023

To help locate family members who have left home. The agency offers location service, particularly in marital situations, and provides some preliminary understanding of why a person may have left home. Similar service is offered to missing persons when located.

Florence Crittenton Association of America
608 South Dearborn Street
Chicago, Illinois 60604

To unite in forming an effective and continuing organization; to develop and maintain standards of service; in general, to assist in bringing about a greater understanding of factors relating to unmarried mothers and adolescent girls with other problems in adjustment.

Lions International
York and Cermak Roads
Oak Brook, Illinois 60521

Community betterment with main objective service to the visually handicapped; provides glasses, cornea bank, seeing eye dogs, and so on.

Mental Health Materials Center, Inc.
419 Park Avenue South
New York, New York 10016

To develop new audiences and new distribution techniques for selected outstanding printed and audiovisual education materials in the fields of mental health, family life, and human relations.

Muscular Dystrophy Associations of America
810 Seventh Avenue
New York, New York 10019

National voluntary health agency dedicated to the scientific conquest of neuromuscular diseases through basic and applied research into nerve and muscle metabolism.

National Association of the Deaf, Inc.
2495 Shattuck Avenue
Berkeley, California 94720

To improve, develop, and extend schools for the

deaf throughout the world, especially in the United States; to eliminate unjust liability, compensation, and traffic laws; to establish state and national labor bureaus for the deaf and all other agencies pertinent to their economic and social welfare.

National Association for Mental Health, Inc.
1800 North Kent Street
Arlington, Virginia 22209

Devoted exclusively to the fight against mental illness. Sponsors and finances research; works for improvement of mental health hospitals; offers communities help in setting up clinics, counseling, and guidance services; rehabilitation programs; helps relatives understand.

National Association for Retarded Children, Inc.
386 Park Avenue South
New York, New York 10016

A voluntary citizen organization dedicated to improved welfare, education, rehabilitation, recreation, health services, and opportunity for the mentally retarded at all age levels.

National Association of Sheltered Workshops and Homebound Program
5530 Wisconsin Avenue, Suite 955
Washington, D.C. 20015

To compile and distribute useful information to suggest and devise standards of operation in the workshop field; to study and make available details of pertinent legislation; to explore the problems of manufacturing and marketing and to interpret and promote better cooperation among private, state, and federal agencies.

National Association of Training Schools and Juvenile Agencies
Glen Mills, Pennsylvania 19342

To provide an open forum for discussion; to promote research; to disseminate information; to encourage training opportunities; to promote cooperation with other organizations having allied interests; and to promote better public understanding toward socially maladjusted children and agencies dealing with them.

National Clearinghouse for Drug Abuse Information
Box 1701
Washington, D.C. 20013

Educational and informational materials related to drug use and abuse are provided for professional and lay groups.

National Cystic Fibrosis Research Foundation
3379 Peachtree Road, N.E.
Atlanta, Georgia 30326

A national nonprofit health organization that since 1961 has set up thirty cystic fibrosis care, research, and teaching centers throughout the country. The foundation is developing local diagnostic and treatment clinics affiliated with the centers.

The National Foundation—March of Dimes
1275 Mamaroneck Avenue
White Plains, New York 10605

Seeks to improve the level of care for all patients with arthritis and birth defects by national grant support of clinical study centers throughout the United States. Grants are made to teaching institutions to conduct clinical research and teaching and to provide patient care.

The National Foundation for Sudden Infant Death
1501 Broadway
New York, New York 10036

Research programs are sponsored by funds contributed; services and information are provided by professionals and parents to parents and families.

National Hemophilia Foundation
25 West 39th Street
New York, New York 10018

A national voluntary health organization dedicated to finding a cure for hemophilia and, until such a cure can be found, to facilitate the management and control of the disease so that hemophiliacs can live normal full and productive lives.

National Rehabilitation Association, Inc.
1522 K Street, N.W.
Washington, D.C. 20005

Promotion in all practical ways of a complete program of rehabilitation for all physically and mentally handicapped persons, and the professional improvement of workers with handicapped persons.

National Society for Autistic Children
169 Tampa Avenue
Albany, New York 12208

To study causes and treatment of autism; services are provided for children and families.

National Society for Crippled Children and Adults, Inc.
2023 West Ogden Avenue
Chicago, Illinois 60612

To carry out the following three-point program: (1) education of the public, professional workers, and parents; (2) research to provide increased knowledge of the causes of handicapping conditions and their prevention and of improved methods of care, education, and treatment; and (3) direct services for crippled children and adults in the fields of health, welfare, education, recreation, rehabilitation, and employment; also to charter and develop state and territorial societies to implement the program at state and local levels.

National Society for the Prevention of Blindness, Inc.
79 Madison Avenue
New York, New York 10016

To study causes of blindness or impaired vision; to advocate measures leading to the elimination of such causes.

National Tuberculosis Association, Inc.
1790 Broadway
New York, New York 10019

To study tuberculosis and other respiratory diseases and to disseminate information and stimulate the programs of its 2,000 affiliated state and local associations for the prevention, treatment, and control of tuberculosis and other respiratory diseases.

North American Association of Alcoholism Programs
1101 15th Street, N.W.
Washington, D.C. 20005

To provide a medium for the exchange of ideas and information regarding organization, policies, and methods relating to state, provincial, territorial, and District of Columbia programs on alcoholism.

President's Committee on Employment of the Handicapped
Washington, D.C. 20203

To provide a continuing program on a day-to-day basis of public information and education designed to provide increased employment of the handicapped in productive tax-paying jobs, free of public or private assistance; to achieve through promotion and voluntary cooperation among its members a maximum of gainful employment and economic security for the handicapped.

President's Committee on Juvenile Delinquency and Youth Crime
Department of Justice, Room 5119
Washington, D.C. 20537

To review, evaluate, and promote the coordina-

tion of activities in the federal government that relate to juvenile delinquency; to stimulate experimentation, innovation, and improvement in federal programs.

Save the Children Federation, Inc.
48 Wilton Road
Westport, Connecticut 06880

To help eliminate the causes of poverty among children in the United States and overseas while maintaining efforts to ameliorate the effects of poverty in those areas where the needs are greatest.

TAISSA (Travelers Aid and International Social Services Association)
345 East 46th Street
New York, New York 10017

To assist youth and adults with problems related to travel, including returning to former residence, assistance in obtaining employment, counseling for personal problems.

United Cerebral Palsy Associations, Inc.
66 East 34th Street
New York, New York 10016

To promote research through a grant program; treatment, education, and rehabilitation of persons with cerebral palsy; to subsidize through grants in aid professional training programs of all types related to the problem of cerebral palsy; to further, by professional and public education, information concerning all aspects of the problem of cerebral palsy; to promote better techniques and facilities for the diagnosis and treatment of persons with cerebral palsy; to act as a source of information on law and legislation in the field of the handicapped, including those disabled by cerebral palsy; to cooperate with governmental and private agencies concerned with the welfare of the handicapped.

Vocational Rehabilitation Administration
Department of Health, Education, and Welfare
Washington, D.C. 20203

To assist states in developing and providing vocational rehabilitation services to help physically and mentally handicapped persons achieve the independence and dignity associated with productive employment.

CHAPTER 10

Assessment tools
and case audit guide

The following assessment tools are presented as suggested guidelines for comprehensive nursing assessment of families and children and for audit of nursing records to determine the quality of care. Included in this chapter are:

Family assessment tool, pp. 129-131
Infant assessment tool, pp. 132-137
Child assessment tool, pp. 138-146

Play assessment tool, pp. 147-149
Case audit guide, pp. 150-151

Completed examples of the use of these tools, as well as the identification and planning for specific health needs and problems, are found in the Unit Cases presented in *Child Health Maintenance: Concepts in Family-Centered Care*.

FAMILY ASSESSMENT TOOL*

I. General data

Number of members in the family:

Stage of development of the family:

Members not living in the household:

Household space and privacy arrangements:

Description of the home environment:

Income: How do you manage to make ends meet?

Transportation available:

Child care arrangements:

Emergency resources:

Eating patterns:

Leisure activities:

Adult friends and relationships outside of family:

Time spent with friends:

Community activities and organizations:

II. Adult social history

Adult relationships as defined within the family:

How adult relationships were formed:

What they consider to be best about their relationship:

What they consider to be worst about their relationship:

*Adapted from Prenatal family assessment tool developed by Kaiser, P., and Kern, D., Texas Woman's University, Dallas, Texas, 1977.

What was life like for you as a child growing up?

Any losses before the age of 15:

As a child, what practice did your parents use in discipline?

What things did you enjoy as a child?

III. **Family interactions** (complete for each family member)

Identity within family:

General health status:

Role in family:

Family tasks:

Life events in previous year:

Previous coping mechanisms:

Developmental state:

Expectations of self:

Expectations of family:

Description of child-adult relationships:

Perception of how decisions are made:

Perceptions of how problems and conflicts are solved:

IV. **Child-rearing**

How do you correct the child when he/she misbehaves?

How do you reward the child for good behavior?

What do you agree that the child should learn in life?

On what do adult members disagree regarding child-rearing?

How do you think the child responds to your discipline/guidance/control?

When do you feel closest to the child?

When do you feel the most distant/strange to the child?

Adult description of each child, including developmental stage and anticipation of events of the coming year:

V. Summary of family's communication

Clarity of speech:

Topic changes/consistency:

Ratio of agreement/disagreement between members:

Intensity of feelings conveyed:

Speaking order:

Commitment to family goals:

Patterns of communication:

VI. Summary of family assessment

Level of family functioning
  Stage of maturity:

  Open/closed:

  Degree of individuation:

  Degree of dependency:

Family strengths:

Active or potential problems:

INFANT ASSESSMENT TOOL*

Infant _____ Sex _____ Age _____ Gestational age _____

Date _____ Race _____

Mother profile

PRESENT HEALTH STATUS:

PRIOR MEDICAL-SURGICAL EVENTS:

PRENATAL HISTORY WITH THIS CHILD

Medical supervision:

Prenatal classes:

Nutrition and diet:

Illnesses, infections, complications:

Treatments and procedures:

Describe your reaction when you first felt the baby move.

Planned or unplanned pregnancy?

Describe home preparations made for the new baby.

Describe how bringing home a new baby will change the life of each member of the family.

Helping persons available:

Named the baby?

LIFE CHANGE EVENTS (DATES)

Death (family, close friend) _____ New baby _____

Divorce _____ Marital separation _____ Return to school _____

Injury, illness _____ Retirement _____ Change of residence _____

PEDIGREE (include chronic, inherited conditions, allergies, causes of death, illness in siblings)

_____

*By Hundley, C., 5122 Alcott, Dallas, Texas 75206, copyright 1977.

O = Female
□ = Male
? = Unknown

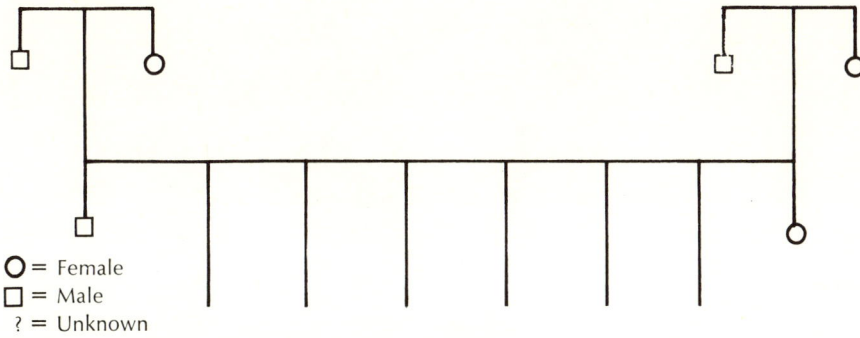

COURSE OF LABOR AND DELIVERY

Duration:

Type of delivery:

Medications and anesthesia (types, durations, reactions, satisfaction with):

Episiotomy:

Fluids–blood–blood loss:

Attended by significant other:

Held and/or nursed baby on delivery table:

FATHER/MOTHER–INFANT INTERACTION

Father/mother:
   Touches infant_____
   Touching pattern, what parts of hands used, where she touches infant:

   Eye-to-eye contact between them:

   High-pitched voice_____
   Entrainment_____
   Holding and feeding positions:

   State of alertness of infant:

Infant profile

NEONATAL STATUS

Risk_____

Apgar_____

Abnormalities:_____

Wt _____ Ht _____ Head circum _____ Chest circum _____

Nutrition:

Medications:

PSYCHOLOGIC PROFILE

Sensory motor   Comments

_____Turns head toward sound outside of vision

_____Searches for sound with eyes

_____Infant watches hand in front of eyes

_____Follows a slowly moving object or face with eyes

_____Stops ongoing activity in response to vocalizations

_____Infant gets hand into mouth; can reinsert if examiner removes

_____Follows disappearing object to point of disappearance

_____Crying

_____Sucking

_____Variations of breathing pattern and change of activity

Trust vs. mistrust   Comments

_____Enjoys eating, sucking activity

_____Follows voices and eyes

_____Relaxed mother-infant interaction

_____Able to sleep after feeding and handling by mother

_____Infant quiets in mother's presence during feeding, changing, holding, comforting

SOCIAL PROFILE

See Father/mother–infant interaction.

Position of child in family:

Life-style of family:

Pattern of family visits to mother and nursery:

Other caretakers for the baby:

ENVIRONMENTAL PROFILE

Space for infant:

Number of people in the home:

Population density:

Infestations:

Fire hazards:

Medications/poisons:

Crime:

Availability of transportation:

PHYSICAL PROFILE

Measurements

Head _____ Chest _____ Wt _____ Ht _____

Gestational age _____

Vital signs _____

Neuromuscular system

Posture, muscle tone (recoil, strength):

Activity level, states of alertness:

Cry/vocalizations:

Reflexes:

Babinski _____	Sucking _____
Plantar _____	Rooting _____
Stepping _____	Moro _____
Crawling _____	Tonic neck _____
Hand grasp _____	Fencing _____
Landau _____	Incurvation of trunk _____

Skin

Color (cyanosis, jaundice, pale, pink):

Texture (dryness, turgor):

Presence of:
    Milia_____
    Vernix (color)_____
    Lanugo_____
    Erythema toxicum_____
    Mongolian spots _____
    Ecchymosis, petechiae, edema

Head
    Fontanels (size, pressure):

    Suture lines/molding:

    Shape of head (caput, cephalhematoma):

    Face (symmetry):

    Eye (scleral hemorrhage, discharge, red reflex):

    Ear (shape, set, amount of cartilage):

    Nose (patency, flaring, discharge):

    Mouth (gums, precocious teeth, Epstein's pearls, palate):

Neck (mobility, edema, openings):

Chest (clavicles, engorgement, excursions, symmetry, nipples):

    Lungs (movement, auscultatory sounds):

    Heart (PMI, murmurs, size, pulses):

Abdomen (contour, bowel sounds, liver, spleen, umbilicus, femorals):

Urinary (location of meatus, characteristics of urine and voiding):

Genitalia (labial swelling, descended testes, spadias, hernias):

Rectum/anus (patency, stools):

Back and spine:

Extremities (palmar creases, ROMs, hip abduction):

CHILD ASSESSMENT TOOL*

I. Client _____ Date _____

Age _____ Race _____ Sex _____ Information _____

II. Reason health care worker sought client:

Reason for seeking health care (mother and child's comments):

What events led up to the situation?

When did this situation occur?

Describe the situation and/or how you are feeling. What made you decide to seek health care?

What do you and your family do when something like this happens?

How is this affecting you and your family at the present time?

III. Family profile

MOTHER

Present health status:

Previous medical-surgical events:

Prenatal history with this child

Medical supervision:

Nutrition, diet:

Illness, infections, complications:

Treatments, procedures:

Anesthesia:

Course of labor and delivery:

Availability in home:

_____

*By Hundley, C., 5122 Alcott, Dallas, Texas 75206, copyright 1978.

Number of people in the home:

Employment/work environment:

Date of last menstrual period:

FATHER

Present health status:

Previous medical-surgical events:

Number of people he supports:

Availability in home/work habits:

Employment/work environment:

Range of income:

Insurance:

Life change events (include dates):

Death (family, close friend) _____ New baby _____ Job loss _____
Divorce _____ Marital separation _____ Return to school _____
Injury, illness _____ Retirement _____ Change of residence _____

Pedigree (include chronic, inherited conditions, allergies, causes of death, illness in
   siblings)

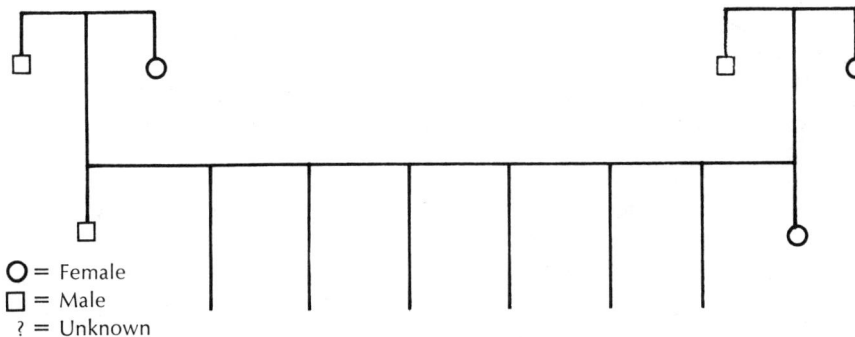

O = Female
□ = Male
? = Unknown

Does your family see itself as a healthy family or as a sick family?

IV. Child profile

NEONATAL STATUS (risk, Apgar, congenital abnormalities):

Postnatal course:

Previous illnesses (dates):

Medications:

Accidents and injuries (dates):

Nutrition history: relate an example of a 24-hour intake:

BFK   LUNCH   SUPPER   SNACKS

Food groups: Meats (2) _____ Veg. (4) _____ Fruit _____
              Breads/cereals (4) _____ Milk/products (3) _____
Formula (type/amount):

Compare weight/height/age ratio:

Identify developmental milestones (DDST):

Sleep patterns/disturbances:

Allergies:

Immunizations:

PSYCHOLOGIC PROFILE (data here to be obtained during interactions, inquiry, observation, DDST)

COGNITION	EGO
Sensory-motor phase (0-24 mos)	Trust vs. mistrust (0-12 mos)
_____ Use of reflexes (early 0-1 mos)	_____ Enjoys eating, sucking activities
_____ Voluntary repetition of reflexes in response to stimuli	_____ Follows voice and eyes
_____ Reaches for an object	_____ Regular eating, sleeping patterns
_____ Manipulation of objects	_____ Relaxed mother-infant interactions
_____ Experiments with manipulation of objects using learned activities	_____ Reaching out for objects
_____ Imitates action of mother or father	_____ Support of mother by father or a significant other

Concrete operations: pre-conceptual thought (2-4 years)

_____Believes everyone views world as he does

_____Play is chief activity; assigns elements of reality to toys, objects

_____Centering: can identify only one quality of an object

_____Imitates parental model

_____Events judged by outward appearance

_____Unable to perform a completed process in reverse (reversibility)

Concrete operations: intuitive thought (4-7½ years)

_____Still believes everyone views the world as he does

_____Identifies objects as having life or motion correctly

_____Conservation: understands that a thing is essentially the same even though shape and texture are altered

_____Classifies objects by any one of several characteristics

_____Identifies tenses of time: past, present, future

Concrete operations: operational thought (8-11 years)

_____Operational thought: mentally orders and relates the experience to an organized whole

_____Sees events from different perspectives

_____Able to return to starting point of an operation (reversibility)

_____Deduction from simple experiences

Formal operational phase (11-15 years)

_____Uses systematic ways for problem solving (relativity)

_____Uses implications from logical deduction for reasoning

_____Reasons with propositions

_____Thinks beyond his own world and beliefs

Autonomy vs. shame and doubt (12 mos-3 years)

_____Sense of will: "I want," "me," "mine"

_____Collects, hoards

_____Interacts more with father

_____Seeks reassurance from parental model after new self-exploration

_____Plays with a world of small manageable toys

_____Unable to stay in a designated place

Initiative vs. guilt (3-6 years)

_____Cares for own body, toys, pets

_____Observes differences between men and women

_____Interacts more with parents and peers

_____Intrusive behavior; questioning, noisy

_____Rivals with older siblings; solitary play or group play with peers; plays out feelings

_____Identifies with parent of the same sex

Industry vs. inferiority (6-13 years)

_____Concentrates on communication with peers

_____Activities segregated by sex

_____Competitive activities

_____Participates eagerly in learning activities

_____Play: relives real-life situation

_____Identifies with an adult other than a parent

Identity vs. identity diffusion (13-18 years)

_____Secondary sexual characteristics

_____Self-image and how others see him are congruent

_____Making long-range plans for occupation in rudimentary form

_____Seeks contacts with members of the opposite sex

_____"Being against" some of societal establishments

Identity vs. identity diffusion
(13-18 years)—cont'd

_____Expresses some basic philoso-
phy and faith

_____Experiments with various roles;
enjoys music, literature, company of others

_____Peers are center of social
interests

Comments:

School progress

What would you like to tell me about school?

What do you like or dislike most about school?

Talk with parent or teacher about memory.

Tell me: What kind of a student do you think you are?

Perception of self

Self-evaluation: Describe yourself to me.

Tell me things you like about yourself; dislike.

Let's pretend you could change something about yourself. Would you change anything?

Describe how you feel about what's happening to you now.

SOCIAL PROFILE

Personal-social (DDST):

Interaction of child with mother and father:

Eye contact:_____

Touching:

Tone of voice of parent:

Child-parent activities:

Ease of separation:

Position of child in family:

Describe life-style.

Is there more than one language spoken in the home?

ENVIRONMENTAL PROFILE

Pollutants:

Population density:

Infestations:

Fire hazards:

Medications/poisons:

Crime:

Availability of transportation:

REVIEW OF SYSTEMS

General:

Hair and scalp (dandruff, lice, cradle cap, itchiness, hair loss):

Skin (infections, scaling, burns, allergies):

Hematopoietic (anemias, bleeding, bruising):

Eyes (infections, blurred vision, squinting, color blindness):

Ears (infection, discharge, eardrum perforation, foreign objects, wax removals, decreased hearing):

Nose, throat, sinuses (runny nose, colds, decreased smell, foreign body, broken nose, tonsillitis):

Mouth and dentition (dental caries, gingivitis, malocclusion, cleft lip and/or palate):

Respiratory (bronchitis, pneumonia, whooping cough, histoplasmosis, tuberculosis, cough):

Cardiovascular (heart murmurs, cyanosis):

Gastrointestinal (nausea/vomiting, diarrhea, constipation, jaundice, pain, colic, gas, hernias, anorexia):

Genitourinary (frequency, urgency, burning, toilet training, bedwetting, odor, stream):

Reproductive (irritations/rashes, deviations, secondary sexual characteristics):

Neuromuscular (convulsions, headache, imbalance, incoordination, muscle weakness, numbness, tremors, tics):

Psychologic (thumb sucking, fears, masturbation):

PHYSICAL PROFILE

Measurements

Head _____ Chest _____ Ht _____ Wt _____

Vital signs

B/P _____ HR _____ RR _____ Temp _____

Neuromuscular system

Present status:

Social affect:

Speech development:

Reflexes:

Biceps _____ Triceps _____ Brachioradialis _____ Patellar _____ Achilles _____

Babinski _____ Eye _____

Cranial nerves

I (olfactory):

II (optic):

III, IV, and VI (oculomotor, trochlear, abducens):

V (trigeminal):

VII (facial):

VIII (acoustic):

IX, X (glossopharyngeal, vagus):

XI (accessory):

XII (hypoglossal):

Cerebellar function (Romberg, walk heel-toe, run in place, touch tip of nose, copy hand movements, pincer grasp, draw and copy geometric shapes):

Parietal lobe (object identification):

Proprioception (positional sense of toe):

Tactile capacity (cold, two-point discrimination, pin prick):

Skin (scars, lesions, turgor, bruises, moles):

Head (circumference, fontanel measurement, palpation, transillumination):

Face (expression, palpebral fissures, placement of ears, percussion of sinuses, symmetry):

Hair, scalp (hairline, hygiene, distribution):

Nose (potency, discharge, smell):

Mouth and throat (teeth, gums, pharynx, tongue, palates, swallowing, tonsils):

Ears (landmarks, structure, hearing):

Neck (nodes, masses, bruits, ROMs):

Chest (symmetry, excursion, nodes, nipples):

Lungs (breath sounds, fremitus, percussion, duration of inspiration, expiration, rate):

Heart (size, position, PMI, sounds):

Abdomen (size, contour, bowel sounds, umbilicus, liver, spleen, femorals):

Back and spine (structure, symmetry, column curvature):

Extremities (palmar creases, ROMs, hip abduction):

Urinary (position of meatus, characteristics of voiding, appearance of urine):

Genitalia (structure, secondary sexual characteristics):

Anus (structure, function):

PLAY ASSESSMENT TOOL*

I. Client _____ Date _____

  Age _____ Race _____ Sex _____

  Information sources (list persons, records)_____

II. Family profile

  MOTHER

  Name:

  Address:

  Phone:

  Marital status:

  Employment (hours, place, days off):

  Educational level:

  FATHER

  Name:

  Address:

  Phone:

  Marital status:

  Employment:

  Educational level:

  LIFE CHANGE EVENTS (state dates and whether it involves mother and/or father if parents are divorced):

  HX OF ILLNESSES (chronic, inherited, allergy):

---

*By Hundley, C., 5122 Alcott, Dallas, Texas 75206, copyright 1978.

SIBLINGS

Number:

Names:

Caretakers:

School:

III. Child profile

Address:

Present health status:

Prior accidents, injuries, illnesses (dates):

Nutritional status:

Weight/height/age ratio:

Developmental milestones appropriate to age:

Sleep patterns/disturbances:

Allergies/medications:

Immunizations:

Nursery school information

Hours at school:

Number of days:

Special precautions/instructions:

SOCIAL PROFILE

Interactions with parent; with teachers; with other children:

Eye contact:

Touching:

Position in the family (birth order):

Languages spoken in the home:

Life-style:

Additional data:

PLAY EXPERIENCE

Time allowed _____ Time used _____

Limits (responsibilities of the child, use of materials, behavioral guidelines):

Theory or concept to be tested:

Setting (materials, environment, controlled variables):

Purpose of the experience:

Special considerations (language level, use of touch, developmental level, maturational level, cultural background):

Description and assessment of the experience:

Suggestions for future planning and intervention:

CASE AUDIT GUIDE

Instructions: After review of a selected case, answer the following questions and cite the evidence that is found in the record.

I. Application of the framework of child competencies
A. Does the record contain assessment data related to physical, learning and thought, social, and inner competencies?
B. Do the assessment data support the conclusions that are made regarding the child's stage of development?
C. What additional information is needed for each competency?
D. Does the plan provide for future acquisition of needed data?

II. Achievement of the nursing process
A. 1. Are the values of the child/adult client and the nurse acknowledged in relation to the needs of the client?
   2. Is the child/adult client involved in identification of problems and planning for care?
   3. Is the nurse an advocate for the child/adult client?
B. 1. Is the structure needed for goal attainment identified, including personnel, monetary resources, and physical facilities?
   2. Is the process or the actions needed to achieve health care goals identified?
   3. Are the outcomes or goals of health care described in measurable or observable terms?
C. 1. Are baseline data or initial health status reported in relation to each health care goal?
   2. Is progress toward goal attainment reported?
D. 1. Are the data obtained interpreted in relation to developmental norms?
   2. Are the data obtained interpreted in relation to cultural values of the family?
   3. Is the interpretation of health needs, health problems, and nursing diagnoses supported by the available data?
E. 1. Does the record reflect consideration of alternative actions and involvement of the child/adult client in selecting the desired action?
   2. Do the actions selected appear to be defensible based on the available data, or would other alternatives be indicated?
F. 1. Do the actions selected reflect sound professional judgment?
   2. Are the actions selected in accord with the values of the child/adult client?
G. Does the record reflect realistic implementation of actions, accounting for the structure, process, and outcomes needed to achieve health care goals?

III. Use of the problem-oriented record
A. Does the data base support the health needs and problems that are on the health status list?
B. Does the data base include:
   1. Initial statement of the client's reason for seeking health care.
   2. Profile of the child/adult client.
   3. Past history of the child, parents, and family.
   4. Review of physiologic systems.
   5. Physical assessment data.
   6. Psychosocial assessment data.
   7. Results of testing or laboratory data.
   8. Summary of the child's stage of development and health status.
C. Does the initial plan include the following for each problem on the health status list:
   1. Subjective data.
   2. Objective data.
   3. Assessment.
   4. Plan.

D. Are nursing orders included for each client objective?

E. Do the progress notes reflect implementation of the plan and nursing orders?

IV. Quality of care as determined by nursing care standards

Using the Maternal and Child Health Standards of Nursing Practice (see Chapter 2 in *Child Health Maintenance: Concepts in Family-Centered Care)*, determine the following:

A. Which assessment factors are demonstrated in this record?

B. Which assessment factors have not been demonstrated that could have been demonstrated in this record?

C. Based on this evaluation, what recommendations would you make for improvement of this nurse's practice?

APPENDIX

Conversion tables and equivalents

CONVERSION TABLES
Metric system

The units of measurement in the metric system are:

meter (m) for length
gram (g) for weight
liter for capacity or volume

(Note: cubic centimeter [cc] also indicates volume.)

With these units the following prefixes are used:

micro	$^1/_{1,000,000}$ of a unit
milli	0.001 ($^1/_{1000}$) of a unit
centi	0.01 ($^1/_{100}$) of a unit
deci	0.1 ($^1/_{10}$) of a unit
deka	10 times the unit
hekto	100 times the unit
kilo	1,000 times the unit
cubic	the total area covered, measured in square lengths

Thus:

1 kilogram (kg) = 1,000 grams (g)
1 gram (g) = 1,000 milligrams (mg)
1 milligram (mg) = 1,000 micrograms (μg)

Avoirdupois and Imperial systems
Weight

1 pound (lb) = 16 ounces (oz)
1 oz = 437.5 grains (gr)

Height

1 yard (yd) = 3 feet (ft)
1 foot (ft) = 12 inches (in)

Capacity

1 gallon = 4 quarts = 8 pints
1 quart = 2 pints
1 pint = 20 fluid ounces
1 fluid ounce = 8 drams (or drachm)
1 dram = 60 minims

Conversion of pounds to kilograms for pediatric weights

Pounds→ ↓	0	1	2	3	4	5	6	7	8	9
0	0.00	0.45	0.90	1.36	1.81	2.26	2.72	3.17	3.62	4.08
10	4.53	4.98	5.44	5.89	6.35	6.80	7.25	7.71	8.16	8.61
20	9.07	9.52	9.97	10.43	10.88	11.34	11.79	12.24	12.70	3.15
30	13.60	14.06	14.51	14.96	15.42	15.87	16.32	16.78	17.23	17.69
40	18.14	18.59	19.05	19.50	19.95	20.41	20.86	21.31	21.77	22.22
50	22.68	23.13	23.58	24.04	24.49	24.94	25.40	25.85	26.30	26.76
60	27.21	27.66	28.12	28.57	29.03	29.48	29.93	30.39	30.84	31.29
70	31.75	32.20	32.65	33.11	33.56	34.02	34.47	34.92	35.38	35.83
80	36.28	36.74	37.19	37.64	38.10	38.55	39.00	39.46	39.91	40.37
90	40.82	41.27	41.73	42.18	42.63	43.09	43.54	43.99	44.45	44.90
100	45.36	45.81	46.26	46.72	47.17	47.62	48.08	48.53	48.98	49.44
110	49.89	50.34	50.80	51.25	51.71	52.16	52.61	53.07	53.52	53.97
120	54.43	54.88	55.33	55.79	56.24	56.70	57.15	57.60	58.06	58.51
130	58.96	59.42	59.87	60.32	60.78	61.23	61.68	62.14	62.59	63.05
140	63.50	63.95	64.41	64.86	65.31	65.77	66.22	66.67	67.13	67.58
150	68.04	68.49	68.94	69.40	69.85	70.30	70.76	71.21	71.66	72.12
160	72.57	73.02	73.48	73.93	74.39	74.84	75.29	75.75	76.20	76.65
170	77.11	77.56	78.01	78.47	78.92	79.38	79.83	80.28	80.74	81.19
180	81.64	82.10	82.55	83.00	83.46	83.91	84.36	84.82	85.27	85.73
190	86.18	86.68	87.09	87.54	87.99	88.45	88.90	89.35	89.81	90.26
200	90.72	91.17	91.62	92.08	92.53	92.98	93.44	93.89	94.34	94.80

Conversion of pounds and ounces to kilograms

Pounds	Kilograms	Ounces	Kilograms	Pounds	Kilograms	Ounces	Kilograms
1	0.454	1	0.028	9	4.082	9	0.255
2	0.907	2	0.057	10	4.536	10	0.283
3	1.361	3	0.085	11	4.990	11	0.312
4	1.814	4	0.113	12	5.443	12	0.340
5	2.268	5	0.142	13	5.897	13	0.369
6	2.722	6	0.170			14	0.397
7	3.175	7	0.198			15	0.425
8	3.629	8	0.227				

Conversion of pounds and ounces to grams

Pounds \ Ounces	0	1	2	3	4	5	6	7	8	9	10	11	12	13	14	15
0	—	28	57	85	113	142	170	198	227	255	283	312	430	369	397	425
1	454	482	510	539	567	595	624	652	680	709	737	765	794	822	850	879
2	907	936	964	992	1021	1049	1077	1106	1134	1162	1191	1219	1247	1276	1304	1332
3	1361	1389	1417	1446	1474	1503	1531	1559	1588	1616	1644	1673	1701	1729	1758	1786
4	1814	1843	1871	1899	1928	1956	1984	2013	2041	2070	2098	2126	2155	2183	2211	2240
5	2268	2296	2325	2353	2381	2410	2438	2466	2495	2523	2551	2580	2608	2637	2665	2693
6	2722	2750	2778	2807	2835	2863	2892	2920	2948	2977	3005	3033	3062	3090	3118	3147
7	3175	3203	3232	3260	3289	3317	3345	3374	3402	3430	3459	3487	3515	3544	3572	3600
8	3629	3657	3685	3714	3742	3770	3799	3827	3856	3884	3912	3941	3969	3997	4026	4054
9	4082	4111	4139	4167	4196	4224	4252	4281	4309	4337	4366	4394	4423	4451	4479	4508
10	4536	4564	4593	4621	4649	4678	4706	4734	4763	4791	4819	4848	4876	4904	4933	4961
11	4990	5018	5046	5075	5103	5131	5160	5188	5216	5245	5273	5301	5330	5358	5386	5415
12	5443	5471	5500	5528	5557	5585	5613	5642	5670	5698	5727	5755	5783	5812	5840	5868
13	5897	5925	5953	5982	6010	6038	6067	6095	6123	6152	6180	6209	6237	6265	6294	6322
14	6350	6379	6407	6435	6464	6492	6520	6549	6577	6605	6634	6662	6690	6719	6747	6776
15	6804	6832	6860	6889	6917	6945	6973	7002	7030	7059	7087	7115	7144	7172	7201	7228
16	7257	7286	7313	7342	7371	7399	7427	7456	7484	7512	7541	7569	7597	7626	7654	7682
17	7711	7739	7768	7796	7824	7853	7881	7909	7938	7966	7994	8023	8051	8079	8108	8136
18	8165	8192	8221	8249	8278	8306	8335	8363	8391	8420	8448	8476	8504	8533	8561	8590
19	8618	8646	8675	8703	8731	8760	8788	8816	8845	8873	8902	8930	8958	8987	9015	9043
20	9072	9100	9128	9157	9185	9213	9242	9270	9298	9327	9355	9383	9412	9440	9469	9497
21	9525	9554	9582	9610	9639	9667	9695	9724	9752	9780	9809	9837	9865	9894	9922	9950
22	9979	10007	10036	10064	10092	10120	10149	10177	10206	10234	10262	10291	10319	10347	10376	10404

Approximate metric and Imperial equivalents

Metric	Imperial	Metric	Imperial
30 g	1 oz	30 mg	½ gr
15 g	½ oz	20 mg	⅓ gr
8 g	120 gr	15 mg	¼ gr
4 g	60 gr	10 mg	⅙ gr
2 g	30 gr	7.5 mg	⅛ gr
1 g	15 gr	6 mg	¹⁄₁₀ gr
600 mg	10 gr	3 mg	¹⁄₂₀ gr
450 mg	7½ gr	1 mg	¹⁄₆₀ gr
300 mg	5 gr	(1,000 μg)	
250 mg	4 gr	0.6 mg	¹⁄₁₀₀ gr
200 mg	3 gr	0.5 mg	¹⁄₁₂₀ gr
150 mg	2½ gr	0.3 mg	¹⁄₂₀₀ gr
100 mg	1½ gr	0.2 mg	¹⁄₃₀₀ gr
60 mg	1 gr	0.1 mg	¹⁄₆₀₀ gr
50 mg	¾ gr		

Useful approximate metric and imperial equivalents:

1 cm = 0.39 inches	1 in = 2.54 cm
1 meter = 1.1 yards	1 ft = 30.48 cm

To convert centimeters to inches:
Divide the length in centimeters by 2.54.
EXAMPLE: The average newborn infant measures 50.8 cm:

$$\frac{50.8}{2.54} = 20 \text{ inches}$$

To convert inches to centimeters:
Multiply the length in inches by 2.54.
EXAMPLE: The average newborn infant measures 20 inches:

$$20 \times 2.54 = 50.8 \text{ cm}$$

Conversion of inches to centimeters

Inches	Centimeters	Inches	Centimeters
10	25.40	17½	44.45
10½	26.67	18	45.72
11	27.94	18½	46.99
11½	29.21	19	48.26
12	30.48	19½	49.58
12½	31.75	20	50.80
13	33.02	20½	52.07
13½	34.29	21	53.34
14	35.56	21½	54.61
14½	36.83	22	55.88
15	38.10	22½	57.15
15½	39.37	23	58.42
16	40.61	23½	59.69
16½	41.91	24	60.96
17	43.18		

Approximate weight equivalents

Apothecary	Metric	Apothecary	Metric
¹⁄₃₂₀ gr	0.2 mg	½ gr	32.0 mg
¹⁄₂₁₀ gr	0.3 mg	¾ gr	50.0 mg
¹⁄₁₆₀ gr	0.4 mg	1 gr	65.0 mg
¹⁄₁₀₀ gr	0.65 mg	1½ gr	0.1 g
¹⁄₆₄ gr	1.0 mg	2 gr	0.13 g
¹⁄₃₂ gr	2.0 mg	2½ gr	0.16 g
¹⁄₁₆ gr	4.0 mg	3 gr	0.2 g
¹⁄₁₂ gr	5.4 mg	5 gr	0.32 g
¹⁄₁₀ gr	6.5 mg	7½ gr	0.5 g
⅛ gr	8.0 mg	10 gr	0.65 g
⅙ gr	11.0 mg	15 gr	1.0 g
¼ gr	16.0 mg	1 dr	4.0 g
⅓ gr	22.0 mg	1 oz	30.0 g
³⁄₈ gr	24.0 mg		

Approximate volume equivalents

Apothecary	Metric	Apothecary	Metric
1 minim	0.06 ml	80 minims	5.0 ml
1⅝ minims	0.1 ml	2 fl dr	7.5 ml
3 minims	0.18 ml	2¾ fl dr	10.0 ml
5 minims	0.3 ml	4 fl dr	15.0 ml
8 minims	0.5 ml	5½ fl dr	20.0 ml
10 minims	0.6 ml	1 fl oz	30.0 ml
12 minims	0.75 ml	1⅔ fl oz	50.0 ml
15 minims	0.9 ml	2 fl oz	60.0 ml
16 minims	1.0 ml	3⅜ fl oz	100.0 ml
20 minims	1.2 ml	4 fl oz	120.0 ml
30 minims	1.8 ml	8 fl oz	240.0 ml
50 minims	3.0 ml	12 fl oz	360.0 ml
1 fl dr	3.7 ml	1 pt	480.0 ml
65 minims	4.0 ml		

Capacity (volume) equivalents

Useful approximate metric and imperial equivalents
1 liter   = 1.75 pints
1 oz   = 30 ml
1 pint   = 0.568 liters or 568 ml
1 gallon = 4.55 liters

Conversion table

Liters		Pints
0.28	0.5	0.88
0.57	1	1.75
1.14	2	3.50
1.70	3	5.28
1.28	4	7.04
2.85	5	8.80
3.42	6	10.50
3.99	7	12.30
4.55	8	14.08

To read the table: 3 liters = 5.28 pints
3 pints = 1.70 liters

Household measurements

	Apothecary	Metric
1 teaspoon	1 dram	4 ml
1 tablespoon	½ fl oz	15 ml
1 teacup	4 oz	120 ml
1 tumbler	8 oz	240 ml

Temperature equivalents

Centigrade	Fahrenheit	Centigrade	Fahrenheit
34.0	93.2	39.0	102.2
34.2	93.6	39.2	102.5
34.4	93.9	39.4	102.9
34.6	94.3	39.6	103.2
34.8	94.6	39.8	103.6
35.0	95.0	40.0	104.0
35.2	95.4	40.2	104.3
35.4	95.7	40.4	104.7
35.6	96.1	40.6	105.1
35.8	96.4	40.8	105.4
36.0	96.8	41.0	105.8
36.2	97.1	41.2	106.1
36.4	97.5	41.4	106.5
36.6	97.8	41.6	106.8
36.8	98.2	41.8	107.2
37.0	98.6	42.0	107.6
37.2	98.9	42.2	108.0
37.4	99.3	42.4	108.3
37.6	99.6	42.6	108.7
37.8	100.00	42.8	109.0
38.0	100.4	43.0	109.4
38.2	100.7		
38.4	101.1		
38.6	101.4		
38.8	101.8		

To convert centigrade to Fahrenheit:
$9/5 \times$ temperature $+ 32$
EXAMPLE: To convert 40° centigrade to Fahrenheit

$$9/5 \times 40 = 72 + 32 = 104° \text{ Fahrenheit}$$

To convert Fahrenheit to centigrade:
(Temperature $- 32) \times 5/9$
EXAMPLE: To convert 98.6° Fahrenheit to centigrade

$$98.6 - 32 = 66.6 \times 5/9 = 37° \text{ centigrade}$$

References and additional resources

Barness, L. A.: Manual of pediatric physical diagnosis, ed. 4, Chicago, 1972, Year Book Medical Publishers.

Chinn, P. L.: A relationship between health and school problems; a nursing assessment, J. Sch. Health **43**:85, Feb. 1973.

Christakis, G., editor: Nutritional assessment in health programs, Am. J. Public Health [Suppl] **63**:1-82, Nov. 1973.

Cooke, R. E., editor: The biological basis of pediatric practice, New York, 1968, McGraw-Hill Book Co.

Fomon, S. J.: Infant nutrition, ed. 2, Philadelphia, 1974, W. B. Saunders Co.

Francis, G. M., and Munjas, B. A.: Manual of socialpsychologic assessment, New York, 1976, Appleton-Century-Crofts.

Green, M., and Haggerty, R. J., editors: Ambulatory pediatrics II, Philadelphia, 1977, W. B. Saunders Co.

Haynes, U.: A developmental approach to casefinding, Washington, D.C., U.S. Department of Health, Education, and Welfare, PHS publication #2017-1969.

Hubbard, C. W.: Family planning education; parenthood and social disease control, ed. 2, St. Louis, 1977, The C. V. Mosby Co.

Hughes, J. G.: Synopsis of pediatrics, ed. 4, St. Louis, 1975, The C. V. Mosby Co.

Klaus, M. H., and Kennell, J. H.: Maternal-infant bonding, St. Louis, 1976, The C. V. Mosby Co.

Krugman, S., and Ward, R.: Infectious diseases of children, ed. 6, St. Louis, 1977, The C. V. Mosby Co.

Maier, H. W.: Three theories of child development, New York, 1969, Harper & Row, Publishers, Inc.

A model act providing for consent of minors for health services, Report of the Committee on Youth of the American Academy of Pediatrics, Pediatrics **51**:293, Feb. 1973.

Paine, R.: Neurologic examination of infants and children, Pediatr. Clin. North Am. **7**(3):471-509, 1960.

Prior, J. A., and Silberstein, J. S.: Physical diagnosis; the history and examination of the patient, ed. 3, St. Louis, 1969, The C. V. Mosby Co.

Ray, O. S.: Drugs, society, and human behavior, ed. 2, St. Louis, 1978, The C. V. Mosby Co.

Riehl, J. P., and Roy, C.: Conceptual models for nursing practice, New York, 1974, Appleton-Century-Crofts.

Rudolf, A. M.: Pediatrics, ed. 16, New York, 1968, Appleton-Century-Crofts.

Schell, P. L., and Campbell, A. T.: POMR—not just another way to chart, Nurs. Outlook **20**:510-514, Aug. 1972.

Shaefer, C., editor: The therapeutic use of child's play, New York, 1976, Jason Aronson, Inc.

Shirkey, H. C., editor: Pediatric therapy, ed. 5, St. Louis, 1975, The C. V. Mosby Co.

Uzgaris, I. C., and Hunt, J. McV.: Assessment in infancy, Urbana, Ill., 1976, University of Illinois Press.

Vaughan-Wrobel, B., and Henderson, B.: The problem-oriented system in nursing, St. Louis, 1976, The C. V. Mosby Co.

Whipple, D. V.: Dynamics of development; euthenic pediatrics, New York, 1966, McGraw-Hill Book Co.

Williams, S. R.: Nutrition and diet therapy, ed. 2, St. Louis, 1972, The C. V. Mosby Co.

DATE DUE

MAR 2 4 1983			
MAR 1 4 1983			